HOME ENCYCLOPEDIA

by
"DIOCLES"

(Diocles is the pen name of a team of Doctors, leading
Consultants, and laymen with special knowledge of medical writing,
who mostly prefer to remain anonymous. The publishers acknowledge
their debt to Dr. David Ryde for the hypnosis section, and to the
Chief Editor who spent many months in writing and research.)

PAPERFRONTS
ELLIOT RIGHT WAY
BOOKS
KINGSWOOD SURREY
UK

Made and printed in Great Britain by
Hunt Barnard Printing Ltd., Aylesbury, Bucks.

CONTENTS

FOR EMERGENCIES, SEE OVERLEAF

List of Illustrations

EMERGENCY INDEX

INTRODUCTION

Men and women are often confused by medical terms. A pain in your back may not seem much until you learn to your horror that you have a "sub-acute interstitial myositis" and begin to wonder how soon the undertaker will be needed. The pain is no more serious whether it be called backache, lumbago or the title above; but medical terms often give rise to unnecessary alarm. One purpose of this book is to explain the more common medical labels in simple language.

Secondly, there is the question of what you can do, as a layman, about a number of illnesses which may come your way. If in any doubt you must consult your doctor. It takes about six years to train a doctor, and even if this book were twenty times as long it would be impossible to include all the knowledge required to treat even the common illnesses; and more often than not, it is dangerous for the layman to try to do so. But doctors are busy people, and you can help yourself and your doctor considerably by knowing what to do about a number of trivial complaints, what to do in an emergency before the doctor calls, and things you can do when you have to nurse a sick person at home. The main purpose of this book is to answer these questions for you.

Medical knowledge is expanding. Troubles which were incurable years ago can now be treated or helped. Unpleasant old treatments may give place to simpler methods. Surgical operations become ever more effective and safe.

It is important for those with chronic illnesses not to give up hope. The advance you need may be about to materialise, so keep in touch with your doctor or Medical Centre.

LOOK IN THE INDEX FOR ANY ILLNESS NOT LISTED ALPHABETICALLY AS THE ITEM MAY BE MENTIONED AS PART OF ANOTHER COMPLAINT.

NOTE: Where suitable medicines are mentioned please note that space prevents naming all equivalent preparations which may be equally good. No slur is intended where a particular one which your doctor may prefer happens not to be the example we give.

HEALTHY LIVING

Prevention is better than cure. Modern knowledge, especially public health measures, have taught us how to prevent many diseases, and if this knowledge were generally applied to our everyday life the health of the community would be improved. Unfortunately, modern conditions are often in conflict with the ideal of healthy living. Even so, much can be done to assist our bodies to remain healthy, and so give them every chance in any fight against disease.

The human body is an extremely delicate mechanism. To work efficiently it requires a constant supply of fuel, which must be adjusted to the body's needs; it requires regular rest, and it is a prey to many outside influences – attacks by small living organisms, known as germs (bacteria and viruses), excessive heat or cold, violence, unsuitable atmospheres and other factors. Before discussing disease, I shall try to indicate the chief factors in maintaining health. The rules are simple, so simple that they seem hardly worth stating, yet time and again, as a doctor, one sees ill health caused by neglect. Your health is your most precious possession – how precious is often not realised, maybe, until it is almost too late. Guard it.

DIET

Food is the body's fuel, and not only enough but a correct balance between the various types is required to keep the body in health. Broadly speaking, the food we eat can be divided into five categories, which we must look into briefly in order to have some understanding of what is meant by a balanced diet.

a) Carbohydrates

These are sugary and starchy foods whose main purpose is to provide energy for the body. Examples in our daily diet are bread, potatoes and sugar. Starches have to be digested down to sugars before being absorbed into the blood. They then act in the same way as sugar to provide energy. If more carbohydrate is eaten than required for immediate physical activity it is converted to fat.

All foods have a known energy potential usually measured in calories. Sugar can be thought of as "empty calories" as it contains no other vitamins or trace elements. Thus sugar and its derivations – puddings, pastries and sweets, are the main items to cut out in a reducing diet. Honey and fruits which contain mixtures of more healthy *fruit* sugars are suitable alternatives for those with a sweet tooth.

There is no doubt that some unfortunate people put on every excess calorie as fat, while the luckier ones "burn up" surplus supplies. So far we have not found a magic drug to convert the metabolism of the "fatties" into that of the lean, and can only advise dietary restriction to 1,500 calories daily. This, combined with moderate exercise – say a 45-minute brisk walk daily, should give a three pound weight loss per week and can be continued until one's weight comes down to the right figure. A maintenance diet of around 2,000 calories will probably have to be adhered to indefinitely. This is the hard part for those who expect one bout of dieting to cure a life-time's obesity. However this sort of diet is really just a sensible eating programme taking the minimum of carbohydrate and plenty of vegetables, fruit and protein. This small amount of carbohydrate should include a little wholemeal bread daily and a small potato.

The aim in reducing weight is to take the load off the heart and joints and prevent the development of arthritis and heart disease.

b) Fats

Most people are familiar with the various forms such as animal fat, butter, margarine and oils. Fats are also a source of energy, and may contain vitamins (explained later). It is thought that diets low in animal fat and high in polyunsaturated oil, e.g. vegetable oils, "Flora" margarine, etc., may protect against coronary heart disease and it is probably wise to use these.

c) Proteins

The body-building foods. They are vital during the period of growth; and are also necessary in adults, to repair and replace body tissues. Proteins are also required to maintain the body's defence against infection, and for the manufacture of substances to deal with invading germs (antibodies). The chief sources of protein in Western diets are meat, fish, poultry, eggs and cheese, although vegetables such as beans contain good protein.

d) Inorganic salts

This term means certain mineral substances which the body cannot do without. Table salt (sodium chloride) which we eat with our meals is one example; and there are others. Calcium and phosphorous are necessary for healthy bones and teeth; the thyroid gland in the neck cannot work well without a sufficient supply of iodine, and iron is required for the manufacture and replacement of the red cells in the blood.

e) Vitamins

These important substances are often misunderstood, being regarded as some kind of "super tonic" to cure all ills. Vitamins are complex chemical substances, used by the body for certain important functions, but required in only tiny amounts. The body cannot carry on without them and, if they are lacking, serious consequences result. Once the body has sufficient of a particular vitamin it cannot use more. There is thus no point in loading the body with vitamins so long as the basic requirements are present. Vitamins are known by letters of the alphabet and the important ones are:–

Vitamin A. Concerned in growth, in defence against infection and in proper functioning of the eye. The results of a shortage are retarded growth in children, an increased liability to infections and several eye conditions including poor night vision (night blindness). Vitamin A is present in butter, eggs, milk and in a number of vegetables and fruits – particularly carrots.

Vitamin B. A group of substances required for a number of

important functions – particularly the healthy working of the brain, nervous system and heart. If lacking, diseases known as beri-beri and pellagra may develop in which these organs are disorganised. These diseases are not common in U.K., but milder shortages of vitamin B may occur especially among the debilitated and old people who for various reasons do not have a sufficiently varied diet. Deficiency of vitamin B_{12} due to poor absorption causes pernicious anaemia. The chief source of the B vitamins is wheat germ, so that wholemeal bread, cereals and oatmeal are valuable. They are also present in yeast extracts, and "Marmite" contains a liberal supply.

Vitamin C. Necessary to keep the blood vessels healthy; if lacking there may be bleeding into the tissues of the body or from the gums (a condition known as "scurvy"). This vitamin occurs in fresh fruits and vegetables particularly those used in salads. It is destroyed by heat so that *overcooked* vegetables are a poor source.

Elderly people are likely to become deficient as they are usually reluctant to eat "hard" fruits such as apples and seem to be less keen on salads than others. Potatoes contain a good supply of Vitamin C just below the skin and may be the most useful source for the elderly if peeled finely or cooked in their jackets. Fruit juices such as "Ribena" or Vitamin C supplements are valuable for the elderly – as for the very young.

Vitamin D. Necessary for the absorption of calcium which is required to keep the bones and teeth healthy. If it is lacking "rickets" may develop, in which the bones become soft and bend. It is present in milk and butter, and is added artificially to margarine. Fish oils, such as cod liver oil, contain Vitamin D in a concentrated form. The recommended dose of these oils *should not be exceeded* as too much Vitamin D can be harmful.

Vitamin E. Seems to be essential for metabolism of fatty acids. It is present in vegetable oils and is never likely to be deficient in the normal Western diet.

Vitamin K. Necessary for the production of one of the blood clotting factors. Deficiency is only likely in new born babies and in liver disease when it can be corrected by injection.

In the U.K. vitamin drops and tablets are available for young children and expectant and nursing mothers at local health clinics.

HEALTH GIVING FOODS

To remain healthy the body requires all the substances mentioned previously in adequate quantities. Nowadays there is considerable anxiety about food additives, the effects of artificial fertilisers, etc. It is too early to know what effects these are having, but in the meantime it is probably wise to eat as much whole food as possible. On the other hand it is foolish to carry this to extremes and, on occasions, convenience meals can make life easier for the harrassed mother.

One mistake in planning a diet is to supply too many carbohydrate foods, which provide energy and temporarily satisfy hunger, at the expense of the other important factors. Most of the important constituents of the diet are contained in milk, eggs, butter, green vegetables, and fresh fruit.

Vegetables and fruit should be eaten daily and many of the vegetables also provide coarse material known as "roughage" or "fibre" which helps to keep the bowels in good order. Fibre is also contained in wholemeal bread, bran breakfast cereals, e.g. "All Bran", and the skins of fruits, which should be eaten whenever possible (the exception is in the case of diverticulitis where your doctor will advise you). Where the skins of fruits cannot be tolerated, powdered bran (available at health food stores) – one or two teaspoons mixed with breakfast cereal – is a valuable source of roughage. Fish provides iodine and calcium, and a fish meal should be eaten at least once a week.

Meat is first-class protein food, which makes it important that a good proportion is used, particularly by growing children. Toddlers and children commonly go through a "food fad" stage. When meat is being refused one of the other protein foods such as milk or eggs can be substituted and these foods can be pleasantly disguised as puddings. Beans are a valuable source of second-class protein and "Baked Beans" are usually enjoyed by children.

Mothers worried about the small quantities of "healthy" foods that their toddlers will eat can usually be reassured that a segment or two of orange, cereal with plenty of milk, a "disguised" egg and baked beans will satisfy the child's nutritional requirements for the day. The less favoured protein foods should continue to be offered without pressure and gradually they will be accepted. In the meantime no harm is done.

Elderly people who have got into a habit of living on refined bread and margarine, cups of tea and biscuits, need to be encouraged to eat extra fresh vegetables, fruit and fruit juice. Dentures can be a problem and dental advice should be sought if mouth problems are interfering with a reasonable diet.

Pulses such as lentils are a good source of second-class protein and although the soya bean receives more publicity as a protein food than the others it is really just another member of this family.

To summarize, use a reasonable amount of protein food, vary your diet as much as possible and include a good measure of fruit and vegetables. By doing so you will not go far wrong.

SLEEP

Sleep is essential, enabling the body to repair the wastages of the day and to replenish energy. People vary in their requirements, but a good working minimum is eight hours for an adult – children need longer, and the elderly need perhaps only five or six hours. Sleeplessness is common, but often due to simple causes. First make sure your bed is comfortable. Expense on a good mattress is well repaid. Bedclothes should be warm but not heavy; in this respect a duvet is useful. Bonuses include easier bedmaking for back sufferers and reduced house dust for asthmatics. The room should be ventilated, never draughty, and as quiet as possible. Try to relax when you go to bed. It is no use taking the worries of the day to bed and expecting sleep. Put your worries aside, make yourself comfortable, and make a conscious effort to relax. For those troubled by sleeplessness, heavy meals and stimulating drinks such as tea or coffee should be avoided at night. Insomnia due to worry can often be cured by getting up, having a biscuit and/or milky drink, and returning to bed more comforted. A long walk late in the evening is a good way of winding down. (Here a dog comes in handy!)

People require less sleep as they grow older and should not worry if they find that they are sleeping less. Winston Churchill is an example of a man who is said to have taken little sleep but nevertheless achieved great things and lived to a great age. An *occasional* sleepless night may be self-treated by a couple of soluble Aspirins or Paracetamol but if bereavement or anxieties are making the sleepless hours a misery, see your doctor who may be able to treat the *underlying cause* or prescribe a *mild non-habit forming sedative*. Too many aspirins can be dangerous. Retired people often like an hour or two's rest after lunch and then stay up later. In some instances worrying over insomnia has a more serious effect than the complaint! See article on INSOMNIA.

EXERCISE

Any machine designed for a particular purpose requires regular use to keep it in good order. The human body is similar, but unfortunately today more and more people use their bodies less and less. Transport takes them to work in the morning; they sit hunched over a desk all day; return home by car or train and collapse into an armchair by the television until bedtime. Is it surprising that under these conditions, their bodies become unhealthy, and a prey to the millions of germs waiting to attack? The energy from food is not required; so, instead of being burnt within the body, a lot of the food is stored up, and the body becomes burdened with increasing quantities of fat. It becomes sluggish so that often a vicious circle is set up. *The less the exercise, the less the inclination to take any and the more flabby and out of condition the body becomes.*

Everyone should aim at some active exercise at least once a day. The city worker could allow extra time on his journey, and walk at least part of the distance to and from work. Advantage should be taken of week-ends and holidays to cultivate an out-of-door hobby such as swimming, open air games if fit, or brisk walking. Short jogs, provided the doctor says you are fit, can help.

Walk like a soldier, head up, chin and tummy pulled in. The hips, to quote Dr. Bill Tucker, a world authority on osteoarthritis, should be kept in the "pinch-proof" buttock position. The knees should be slightly bent so you use your muscles and not your ligaments. Try sometimes to remember these health-creating points. A bout of exercise should last a few minutes only to begin with and be repeated at five minute intervals in half hour sessions. Choose something you enjoy and your tolerance of the effort involved will soon increase.

FRESH AIR

The same conditions which result in too little exercise tend to limit the use of fresh air. An atmosphere may be unsuitable for the body for several reasons. It may contain injurious impurities; despite the Clean Air Act of 1956, the air in towns still contains toxic matter such as sulphur dioxide and lead (from petrol). The air may be too humid, which means that it carries too much water vapour which interferes with the normal working of the sweat glands. It may contain too little oxygen; normally the body uses up oxygen from the air and releases another gas called carbon dioxide. When a large number of people are in a confined space the oxygen tends to become reduced and the carbon dioxide increases.

The other danger which results from overcrowding and underventilation is the spread of germs. These are always present, but the numbers are enormously increased where people are crowded, so that there is a risk of infectious diseases being spread. Nearly everyone will know how a "cold", brought into an office by one person, will spread until nearly all the occupants are affected.

Fresh air is highly desirable from many points of view. Most of us cannot choose our work; but we can at least see that windows are open in the office, and in the trains on which we travel *provided draughts and objections from others are avoided!*

Don't become a fanatic, for draughts can harm, but there should be sufficient ventilation to change the room air many times daily without undue commotion. With babies and the over sixty-fives care should be taken to avoid the room temperature dropping below at least 68°–70°F (20°–21°C). These groups are unable to maintain body temperatures easily and are at risk from hypothermia (body damage caused by overcooling). Nevertheless babies need the benefit of circulating air: they should never be tightly swaddled in several layers of blanket.

SMOKING

Smoking is a form of addiction depending on the sedative effect of nicotine on the brain and nervous system. There is no doubt that cigarette smoking is harmful and that it damages lungs, heart, arteries, eyes and digestive system. The lungs become coated with tar causing shortness of breath, bronchitis and worst of all, lung cancer. Smoking is also an important factor in the development of coronary heart disease and blockage of arteries in the legs. Peptic ulcers are common in smokers and severe defects of vision can occur.

Pipe smoking carries a lower risk, although there is some danger of tongue and lip cancer. Cigars are less harmful and where a cigarette smoker finds that he cannot (will not) break the habit completely, a change to one of these other forms may be useful. Using a low tar brand of cigarette is also worthwhile although not a substitute for giving up the habit. See article on ADDICTION.

HOW TO STOP

For those anxious to give up smoking I do not know any easy road. It is a matter of will-power. The first week without tobacco can be unpleasant, but I think that to cut down gradually only prolongs the agony. The answer is to stop smoking, and to resist the temptation to have "just one" cigarette.

Some find sucking boiled sweets or chewing gum helps during the early stages. After a week or two the urge dies away. It is then easy to do without tobacco provided one is *firm*. Unlike some addictions this one can be abandoned without special treatment because you CAN stop. Having a job where a No Smoking rule applies is useful, as is keeping as busy as possible. Observation indicates that the upper and middle income groups have largely dropped the habit, but greater affluence among lower income people seems to have increased smoking among *them*. The wisest thing is never to start smoking or *never* to inhale.

If one must have something to soothe, limit smoking to social occasions, or make a rule "never smoke before afternoon tea" or "only in the evenings" or "only at parties". (Most local health authorities in the U.K. run anti-smoking clinics and information about these can be obtained from the Local Community Health Office.)

DRINKING

The use of alcohol is widespread in civilised communities. Alcohol is mildly poisonous and therefore the more taken the more injurious it will be. In large quantities over a prolonged period it will cause insidious but permanent damage to the brain, and liver. An occasional social drink is not going to harm or shorten life.

Please reserve alcohol for special social occasions and *do not allow it to become a daily or solitary habit*. Wines are more potent than beer, while spirits such as whisky or gin are highly concentrated and therefore more dangerous. It is, however, possible to get hooked on any of these forms, even the more dilute. Alcohol can get such a grip on an individual that he is unable to do without it, and his health ruined. He will probably need long-term skilled treatment in an attempt to break the addiction.

THE BOWELS

The chief function of the bowels is to eliminate waste matter from the body. This is mostly derived from the food we eat, and the waste products of digestion. Usually, plenty of roughage, bran and fluids should ensure that the bowels work efficiently. Laxatives which in most instances act by "flogging" the bowels should be avoided as far as possible. *Any persistent change in bowel habit needs medical investigation*. It is important for health that the bowels should work normally, and it is common under conditions of civilisation to find that they do not. For those who are troubled consult the article on CONSTIPATION.

GENERAL CONSIDERATIONS

Many important items in healthy living have been considered, but it is obvious that these are not all. Stress is a major factor in the modern way of life. The body is largely under the control of the mind, and if this is not in a settled state, the workings of the body can be upset, and ill health result. It is useless to advise people not to worry. We all have worries, and indeed, life is largely made up of them. The danger lies, not in considering our problems, but in letting them get the upper hand. Don't let your troubles prey on your mind so that you take them to bed with you, re-examine them each morning and finally get into a state where life seems to hold no enjoyment. Keep them under control, and you will find that even serious problems usually develop unexpected turns for the better in time.

If you find that you are constantly ruminating over problems to the detriment of work, sleep or family life, it may be that you need help for an anxiety state. Sometimes talking things over with your spouse or a close friend helps to pinpoint and perhaps reduce the source of stress. If this does not help, you should get your doctor's advice. (*See* ANXIETY STATE.)

Another consideration is one's mental attitude towards health. A man has only one body to last him all his days, and, if it is neglected until past repair, nothing can replace it. The moral is obvious. If you want to remain healthy, do not neglect nature's warnings. Take your body or mind to a doctor for advice as readily as you would take your car to a garage.

It is equally foolish to go the opposite extreme and imagine that every little ache and pain is a major disorder. The body is a delicate piece of mechanism easily upset. We all suffer from temporary upsets of one kind and another, and these are not of great importance, and soon pass. The conditions for which advice should be sought are too numerous to detail, but in general any departure from the normal which *persists*, or *recurs regularly*, should be a warning sign. Thus an occasional headache attacks nearly all of us, but is without special significance. If, however, you were to wake up with a bad headache *every* morning for a week or ten days without apparent cause you would be foolish not to consult your doctor.

Hypochondriacs are people whose illnesses are largely imaginary and in recent years their numbers seem to have increased; make no mistake, they and their families suffer desperately. This may be due in part to increasing medical information propagated by the media where the emphasis is often on catastrophe rather than hope. We deal more fully with this under "Mental Illnesses" and other headings later.

Healthy living is not difficult. Beware of cranks and fads; use a liberal dose of common sense in your daily life, exercise moderation – *even in keeping to the rules*, for nothing is more deadly than boredom, and when in doubt consult an expert – your doctor.

A

Abortion. *(Miscarriage)*

This term is used when a pregnancy ends before the 28th week. After that the condition is known as premature labour. Among lay people the term "miscarriage" is generally used, as "abortion" is usually understood to imply an operation, legal or otherwise.

A few women show a little loss of blood when the first period should be due even though they are pregnant. Apart from this there should be no loss or discharge during pregnancy, and if there is it means that something is wrong and a miscarriage is threatened. When this occurs prompt action is needed if the baby is to be saved.

Sometimes during the first three months, often for no apparent reason, the patient begins to lose a little blood. She may also have some low backache, and complain of feeling generally unwell. She should be put to bed immediately, kept warm, and the doctor called urgently. She may go to the toilet but should be in earshot of help and should not lock the door. Any blood or tissue passed should be kept for the doctor's inspection (a chamber pot or child's "potty" is valuable for this purpose). Internal tampons should be avoided because of the risk of infection. An ordinary "sanitary towel" is better at this time. Often the blood loss stops quite quickly and after a few days' rest at home the patient may be able to resume normal activities. After a threatened miscarriage or a history of repeated miscarriages it is advisable to abstain from intercourse for the first three months of pregnancy.

If the blood loss continues for more than a few days or if contraction pains develop it is likely that the miscarriage will be inevitable. Your doctor will advise you further and arrange for hospital admission if he feels that this is necessary.

Usually after a miscarriage in hospital the uterus (womb) is gently cleared of any remaining tissue so that blood loss is kept to a minimum. Often a woman is advised to avoid pregnancy for a further two or three months but this is variable and many women are fighting fit within a month.

The abortion law was altered in the U.K. in 1967 permitting abortion for certain reasons. Termination of pregnancy is now permissible if the physical or mental health of the mother and her existing family is likely to be adversely affected by its continuing to full term. It is also permissible if there is a substantial risk that the infant will be born with a serious malformation or handicap. A declaration to this effect must be signed by two doctors (one of whom must have specialist qualifications in gynaecology) and the operation must be carried out in a clinic or hospital department approved for the purpose by the Department of Health.

An important cause of abnormality in the new-born baby is the occurrence of German Measles (Rubella) in the mother during the first three months of pregnancy. This is a strong medical indication for termination of pregnancy although of course the mother makes the final choice, bearing in mind the risks.

Although abortion has its opponents, one good effect has been the drastic fall in mortality and ill health following botched illegal operations. No woman in the U.K. should need to consult an unqualified abortionist or consider taking drugs to end an unwanted pregnancy. The risks of an illegal operation carried out under non-sterile conditions include severe haemorrhage, infection leading to peritonitis, subsequent sterility and even death.

Your doctor (or the British Pregnancy Advisory Service) will advise you if you need help in this matter.

Abrasion.
An injury to the outer skin exposing the deeper layers. These grazes are common, especially in children, and are not serious. The chief danger is infection. Minute living organisms (or germs) may get into the tissues where they cause inflammation and pus or "festering". Abrasions should be cleaned with cooled, boiled water to which some antiseptic such as Savlon or Dettol has been added. Where clean water is not available saliva which has some "anti-germ" properties is a useful if crude alternative. ("Suck and

spit".) A small abrasion is best left open to the air to heal. If large, it should be covered with a 'non-stick' dressing (e.g. Melolin) and left for three or four days. If pus develops in spite of this treatment consult your doctor as antibiotics may be needed.

Abscess.

A collection of pus. When germs enter the body there is a fight between them and the body's defences, and pus is usually formed. It contains dead germs, dead blood cells and fluid which has poured into the affected area.

Most abscesses are near the surface, due to germs invading the skin and are usually called boils or carbuncles. Sometimes abscesses form internally following various diseases, for instance in the lung after pneumonia. These are serious matters outside our scope. For the treatment of boils and carbuncles see the appropriate headings.

Achilles' Tendon.

This is the thick tendon at the back of the ankle which can rupture spontaneously. Pain due to rupture feels like a blow at the back of the calf and the patient can only hobble with difficulty using the flat of the foot. Prompt medical treatment is required (usually surgical repair and/or plaster of Paris).

Acidosis.

This term has a precise medical meaning applied to conditions in which the amount of acid in the body, and particularly in the blood, is increased. Often it is used in a wider sense by lay people to cover conditions such as an upset stomach, or vomiting in children. In this sense the condition may be due to excessive eating or drinking, and is best remedied by giving the stomach a rest. A teaspoonful of bicarbonate of soda in a glass of cold water on rising, and light meals for the rest of the day will usually put matters right.

Acne.

A common condition in which the face, and sometimes the upper part of the trunk, is covered with spots. It is caused by blockage and infection of sebaceous or oil glands whose purpose is to lubricate skin and hair. It is most common in teenagers – and is partly due to glandular changes. Treatment is not easy, but cleanliness – frequent but not excessive washing with medicated or tar soap – helps to reduce the number of spots. *Over-enthusiastic cleaning has been found to aggravate the condition in some instances. It is important to avoid squeezing the spots or indeed touching the skin unnecessarily as infection can be spread.*

There are many lotions and creams which can be prescribed by your doctor so no-one need feel downhearted about this condition. Applications include sulphur, cortisone, Vitamin A derivatives and abrasive creams which reduce the thickened skin around large spots. Hair kept well away from the face allows the beneficial effects of sunlight to reach the skin. A diet low in fats, especially chocolate, is usually recommended although some now doubt if this is really necessary. In many cases a fairly prolonged course of antibiotics is needed and this is usually effective as is ultraviolet ray treatment.

Usually the condition clears up as adult life is reached and the self-conscious teenager should be reassured about this.

The contraceptive pill may aggravate acne and any young woman who has or had acne should bear this in mind when considering contraception.

Acupuncture.

Ancient Chinese medical art of inserting fine needles into specific points on the body determined by the patient's symptoms and pulse information.

It is often used for pain relief and anaesthesia and in the West seems to be of most value in treating chronic pain such as neuralgia and low backache. It has also been used for the treatment of drug addiction.

In China major operations are carried out on the conscious patient using acupuncture as anaesthetic. Relaxants and other drugs may be given at the same time.

Western doctors have no complete explanation for the effects of acupuncture although as it seems to be of most use in pain relief it is thought possible that it may interfere with the passage of pain sensations through the various nerve junctions. More likely it is due to psychological conditioning of the patient. Acupuncture will not halt any progressive conditions such as cancer and should not be thought of as an alternative treatment in such diseases.

The Chinese deny the psychological story and among other things claim that the needles help to drain harmful forces from the body to restore the natural balance.

Acute.

Sudden, short-lived e.g. *acute* appendicitis, which requires immediate treatment. The opposite is "chronic" which means long, drawn out. A chronic appendicitis may go on for months with occasional attacks of pain before treatment is decided upon.

Addiction.

An overwhelming desire or need for a drug. This occurs with the "socially acceptable" drugs (alcohol and nicotine) as well as the illegal amphetamines ("speed"), heroin and cocaine. Addiction implies that the body has become physically dependent on the drug and that there will be unpleasant withdrawal symptoms if the drug is stopped.

With most drugs (except perhaps nicotine) eventually the addict becomes obsessed with obtaining his supplies at any cost, to the detriment of his work and family life. The final result is total breakdown of mental and physical health unless specialist treatment can be obtained. Even then, cure is difficult and uncertain. *Only a fool would start such bad habits.* There is nothing clever or brave in experimenting with illegal drugs. (*See* DRUG, DRUG ADDICTION *and* SMOKING, *page 15*.)

Adenoids. *(Mouth breathing)*

Small patches of tissue which grow at the back of the nose. They are part of the body's defence against germs entering through the nose, and are similar to the tonsils which help to guard against germs entering through the mouth. Sometimes, in children, the adenoids become chronically infected and grow so large as to obstruct the nose breathing. When this happens the child speaks with a nasal voice, becomes a mouth breather, and may have frequent purulent discharge from the nose. This may be associated with recurrent ear infections and hearing difficulty due to passage of the germs along the Eustachian tube to the middle ear (see fig. 6 page 87). It is then necessary to remove the adenoids. This is a small operation and the child should be out of hospital in a few days.

The tonsils are sometimes enlarged in such cases and may be removed (see fig. 14 page 216).

Adrenal Glands.

Two small glands situated above the kidneys. They manufacture various substances (hormones) which pass into the blood and help to regulate the workings of the body. One of these, known as *adrenalin*, increases the heart rate and enables the body to act quickly in emergency. Others control many complex bodily functions and are important in coping with stresses such as infection. Disease of the adrenal glands causes a wasting illness known as *Addison's disease*. Sufferers can be helped considerably by cortisone treatment, in which the missing substances, which ought to be manufactured by the adrenals, are supplied artificially.

After Pains.

Pains felt after the birth of the child due to the uterus contracting down to its original non-pregnant size. (*See* CHILDBIRTH.)

Air Sickness. (*See* EARACHE, TRAVEL SICKNESS *and* VOMITING.)

Alcoholism.

Alcoholic drinks have been consumed for centuries. Research disproves that alcohol is a brain stimulant. It damps the higher functions so that we are less self-conscious, less aware of our shortcomings and generally develop a spirit of goodwill towards others. In excess or simply taken regularly, alcohol is habit forming. (*See*

DRINKING (*page 16*) *and* ADDICTION.) To drink excessively is a sign of weakness not strength.

Damage to the liver can occur long before social effects are obvious. Busy young executives involved in business lunches and trips abroad *are frequently surprised to learn that their liver function tests are abnormal on routine testing.*

At this stage, total abstinence can result in the return of liver functions to normal. If the warning is ignored liver damage can become permanent as cirrhosis develops. This condition may be associated with chronic ill health before jaundice, coma and death eventually supervene.

Alcoholism can be said to exist if the drinking habit is having an adverse effect on the work, family or social life of an individual. Specialist help should be urgently sought as the condition is progressive and disintegration of the personality as well as damage to the brain and other systems of the body can occur. The organisation "Alcoholics Anonymous" is a great help to most sufferers and its sister organisation "Al Anon" for the distressed relatives also provides a valuable service.

Delirium tremens (D.T.'s) is a grave condition commonly seem in habitual drinkers, often young. The patient is delirious, trembling and has vivid, unpleasant hallucinations. The condition is so distressing that the patient usually begs for sedation. Frequently there is accompanying heart failure or pneumonia and urgent treatment is required.

Cheap alcohols such as surgical, industrial and methylated spirits are extremely dangerous as they contain "wood alcohol" which can cause blindness and death. Tragedies have occurred among young people at parties where punch has been laced with industrial or methylated spirits; such behaviour is criminal.

Other tragedies have resulted from the drinking of large volumes of *spirits* by young men "for a dare". Death from acute poisoning can occur quickly in these circumstances. It should not be forgotten that even in modest quantities alcohol is *poison*. Also it reacts in combination with certain drugs, causing disasters.

Two or three drinks accompanying plenty of food at an occasional social gathering is quite enough and no-one should mix their drinks.

Allergy.

A condition of abnormal sensitivity of the body to certain outside influences. The sensitivity is usually inherited. Some people are allergic to certain foodstuffs e.g. shellfish, nuts, eggs, etc. In those cases there may be puffy swelling of the face or tongue, or skin rash resembling widespread nettle rash. A similar allergic response can occur with antibiotics, notably penicillin.

In some instances, particularly with reactions to insect stings or drugs, the response may become more marked with each attack so that eventually breathing distress and collapse can occur.

It is important to note and advise your doctor of any unusual reactions to tablets or proven allergies and to avoid these substances. A bracelet engraved with allergy information and indeed any medical data can be obtained (in the U.K.) and may be valuable in emergency when for some reason e.g. loss of consciousness, you are unable to give the information verbally.

Whilst avoiding the offending substance is the best treatment for allergy, there are drugs such as antihistamines, adrenalin, disodium cromoglycate and cortisone which control it.

Injecting minute doses of suspicious substances into the skin can be a useful way of identifying allergens. The information obtained can be used to make up courses of desensitizing vaccines by which regular exposure to gradually increased doses of allergic substances causes reduction of the allergic response. These injections seem to be of use mainly in hay fever and in some cases of asthma.

Alopecia. (*See* BALDNESS)

Amenorrhoea.

Cessation of normal menstruation – the monthly period in women. Periods normally stop some time between the ages of 44 and 54 at the time of the menopause after which the woman is no longer capable of childbearing.

The usual temporary cause of amenorrhoea before this is pregnancy. Many general illnesses, especially if prolonged and debilitating, are associated with absence of the periods, and sometimes a period is missed in a healthy woman for no apparent reason. Worry can also cause amenorrhoea, and a woman may be so worried by the possibility of a pregnancy as to miss a period and thus (so she thinks) confirm her worst fears. A disruption of routine and homesickness can cause missed periods. Nurses, students and new recruits to the women's forces often suffer from this for the first few months. The contraceptive pill causes light and occasionally missed periods.

In the absence of other symptoms one missed period should not be a cause for alarm, but if a second is missed consult your doctor. Less commonly amenorrhoea may indicate that the ovaries are failing to release eggs in the usual way, and occasionally this occurs in some glandular disorders.

Amenorrhoea is also an important symptom in anorexia nervosa (*see* ANOREXIA) and indicates that excessive dieting has disturbed the girl's hormone balance.

Frequent bouts of amenorrhoea in otherwise healthy young women may be associated with subfertility and such patients should probably not use the contraceptive pill which acts by suppressing ovulation.

Amnesia.

Loss of memory. Memory may be lost after head injury and the loss usually covers a variable period before the trauma. In other cases memory loss may be a symptom of mental illness, or stress. The condition calls for expert assessment, but fortunately the memory is usually recovered. Some patients *pretend* to have lost their memories (perhaps to gain attention). (*See* MENTAL ILLNESS.)

Anaemia.

The average human body contains about eight pints of blood, which is pumped round by the heart and nourishes the tissues. A large part of the blood is composed of small particles known as red blood cells. These carry oxygen from the lungs to all the tissues, and this oxygen is necessary to keep them alive. In anaemia the number of red cells (or corpuscles) is reduced and the body is not able to work as it should. The patient is usually pale since the amount of red pigment in the blood is reduced. Sufferers are easily tired, short of breath, and may have headaches and chest pain. Women suffer more than men since their monthly period causes a drain on the red cells. There are many causes of anaemia, but the most common is shortage of iron in the diet, since iron is required for the manufacture in the body of haemoglobin – the pigment contained in the red cells.

In pregnancy there is even more risk of anaemia developing as enough haemoglobin for two must be obtained. The expectant mother needs extra iron as well as folic acid (another essential factor for developing red cells).

Anaemia may also be due to lack of vitamin B_{12}, vitamin C, thyroid hormone and excessive breakdown or loss of red cells. This last occurs in acute haemorrhage or following frequent small bleeds from "haemorrhoids" or "hiatus hernia" (see appropriate headings).

A diet rich in meat, eggs, liver, green vegetables and fresh fruit should correct most mild deficiency states. Supplements of iron and vitamins B and C may help, e.g. ferrous gluconate and multivite tablets each three times a day.

Failure to respond may mean there is a more complex reason for the anaemia and a fuller medical investigation is needed. (*Also see* PERNICIOUS ANAEMIA.)

Anaesthesia.
The abolition of pain during operations, usually by putting the patient to sleep. The substance used is called an *anaesthetic* and nitrous oxide (laughing gas) and halothane are probably the best known. They work by damping down the action of the brain until consciousness is lost, and the patient becomes relaxed. Further relaxation is achieved by the use of muscle relaxant injections. Under these conditions operations can be performed painlessly and easily. Anaesthesia is usually induced by an injection into the bloodstream and maintained by gases.

Minor dental operations can often be performed under intravenous anaesthesia or relaxation without gas. Sometimes injections are made into the nerves of the part to be operated on (local anaesthesia) so that no pain can be felt. The dentist's injection into the angle of the jaw is one type of "nerve block". Similar injections can be made around the lower spinal cord rendering the whole of the *lower* half of the body numb. This type of anaesthesia, known as "epidural", may be used in childbirth. It requires very specialised facilities and not all women wish to have no feeling during such an exciting time.

Many of the benefits of modern surgery are possible only because of the recent improvements in anaesthetics.

Aneurysm.

A weakness in the wall of a blood vessel which causes it to bulge. One type may develop in older people in the large blood vessel (the aorta) which leaves the heart.

Angina Pectoris.

A form of heart disease in which the blood supply to the heart becomes inadequate. As the body ages the blood vessels become harder, and thicken so that they are able to carry less blood. The heart is a muscle which pumps the blood and if the coronary arteries which nourish the heart muscle are hardened the heart cannot work efficiently. When the sufferer attempts something too much for the heart e.g. walking up a hill, a pain (which passes after a short rest) develops in the centre of the chest. Sufferers need medical advice as various medicines including trinitrin and betablockers may help. Their aim is to open up the circulation in the unaffected arteries and reduce the strain on the heart.

The patient can help by giving up smoking, reducing excessive weight, eating a diet low in animal fat and gradually building up physical activity within the limit of his angina. The most suitable exercise to start on is walking on the flat and this may be increased gradually as long as there is no pain. Many people live for thirty years or more after a diagnosis of angina so never feel discouraged and keep moving!

Anorexia Nervosa

A condition usually in young women who diet excessively sometimes with fatal results. It may be difficult to recognise and treat as these girls are adept at concealing their weight and lack of eating. They are not *always* overweight in the first place and although anorexia means literally loss of appetite these patients may be controlling a ravenous appetite with will power. Periods of dieting may alternate with "binges" in which the sufferer gorges secretly and indiscriminately. After a "binge" the girl may induce vomiting by putting her fingers down her throat. Somewhere along the line the periods stop and this is an important symptom of anorexia. The condition is said to represent a failure to come to terms with developing sexuality and the girl often has other symptoms of emotional disturbance. Urgent treatment in a specialist unit is required.

Antibiotics.

Powerful drugs obtained originally from living organisms such as yeasts (several can now be synthesised chemically) for treatment of infections. Penicillin was the earliest; others now often used are derivatives of penicillin, tetracycline and erythromycin. The sulphonamides (the earliest was "M & B") perform a similar function but are not obtained from living tissue and are therefore not strictly speaking anti*biotics*. In the U.K. these are available on prescription only and the course should always be completed.

Antrum.

A hollow in the cheekbone which communicates through a small opening with the nose. The most important hollow spaces in the bones of the skull are the two antra, one in either cheek, and the two sinuses above the eyebrows. Unfortunately, especially after a cold, germs may get into these spaces and set up infection. This results in a chronic discharge from the nose, and pain in the area, a condition known as *sinusitis*. If the antrum is affected there is pain and tenderness in the cheek. If a frontal sinus is affected there is pain above the eyebrows and often a headache on rising which wears off during the day. In this condition the nose must be kept clear to allow the sinus or antrum to drain. Inhalations of the vapour of "Friars' Balsam", one teaspoonful to a pint of boiling water are useful. If the condition does not clear quickly your doctor should be consulted as antibiotics or sinus washout may be required.

Anxiety State.

Persistent feelings of anxiety such as shaky hands, sweating, palpitations, jumpiness and sleep disturbance. There may be no immediately obvious cause or the sufferer may have long-standing family or work problems wit which he can no longer cope. The conditions make it increasingly difficult for the person to solve his problems and medical advice should be sought if talking things over with spouse or close friends does not help. It is *normal* to have anxiety symptoms like shakiness for some hours or days after a severe shock like a narrow escape from a road traffic accident. Thyroid and gland troubles can cause these feelings. (*See* ADRENAL GLANDS, GOITRE *and* MENTAL ILLNESSES.)

Appendicitis.

A disease of civilization. Food passes from the stomach through a long tube (the intestine) which lies coiled inside the abdomen. At one point there is a small side branch, the *appendix,* which comes to a blind end. (*See* FIG. 1.) In lower animals this is larger and has a part to play in digestion, but in man it is probably only rudimentary.

FIG. 1 Contents of the abdominal cavity

A   Liver
B   Gall bladder
C   Duodenum
D   Appendix
E   Spleen
F   Stomach
G   Pancreas
H   Small intestine
I   Colon (large intestine)
J   Bladder

Appendicitis means inflammation of the appendix (all medical terms ending in "-itis" mean inflammation, e.g. cystitis, etc.). Partly-digested food may enter the appendix, and as there are always germs in the intestines, irritation and infection of the appendix may result. This may cause swelling of the appendix, in the same way as the skin round a boil will swell, so that the infected matter is unable to get out of the blind tube. Appendicitis has then developed, and if allowed to continue the appendix may burst and spread the infection over the whole of the inside of the abdomen – causing peritonitis – a grave condition.

Appendicitis usually starts with an aching pain in the centre of the abdomen around the navel, and there may be sickness or a little diarrhoea. More commonly there is constipation. There is usually fever, so that the temperature is raised to 99° to 100°F (about 37½°C); and after a while the pain moves down to the right side, and becomes more severe. The patient should be put to bed and a doctor called, as, if it is appendicitis, treatment is to remove the appendix. A doctor must be contacted early before there is danger of the appendix bursting and spreading the infection. There is one rule that everyone should remember. *In a case of stomach ache, particularly in a child, never give a laxative without a doctor's instruction.* If it is appendicitis the violent action of the bowels caused by the aperient may cause the appendix to burst, with fatal results. If there is no fever and constipation is suspected, a glycerine suppository may be safely given.

Arteries.

The thick-walled blood vessels which carry blood from the heart. After the blood has been distributed to the tissues of the body it is collected in thin-walled blood vessels, *the veins*, which return it to the heart. (*See* HEART DISEASE.)

Arteriosclerosis.

The condition in which the walls of the arteries become thickened and hard.

Such thickening of the coronary arteries causes angina, whilst arteriosclerosis in the legs causes intermittent calf pain on walking. The condition is commonest in smokers, and in those with a tendency to raised blood cholesterol. Smoking should be stopped, and medicines to lower blood cholesterol can be given. A low animal fat diet is probably wise; it has been found that onions and garlic are helpful in reducing blood fats, and this may be useful when drugs are poorly tolerated or unavailable.

Arteritis.

Inflammation of the wall of an artery. An important type is that which occurs in the scalp temple artery as it may be associated with loss of vision. Persistent soreness over the temple area in an (usually) over 65 person requires *urgent* medical advice as treatment (usually steroids) can preserve vision. Failure to treat may result in sudden blindness – usually in one eye. Improvement in lost sight can some-times be restored by a few months of special "non-animal fat" diet, etc. Misdiagnosis can occur in this illness, so a second opinion may be advisable.

Arthritis.

Inflammation of the joints, common in the middle-aged and old. There are many varieties. Sometimes one or more joints are affected during some other illness; e.g. German Measles. This type of acute arthritis usually clears up com-pletely. (*See* ACUTE.) RHEUMATIC FEVER is also associated with acute inflammation of the joints.

The usual types of arthritis, however, are chronic and develop slowly, and may last for years. The commonest form is OSTEOARTHRITIS which can be thought of as a result of "wear and tear". It may also be a late result of injury or fracture. It occurs in the older age groups and commonly in the joints most under stress – such as hips, knees and spine. The joints should remain as mobile as possible and unless they are acutely inflamed and hot – *exercise is vital. It could be said to be so essential that one's future life and enjoyment depend on it.* Normally 10 minutes a day should suffice. In the large joints such as the hip and knee there is a tendency for the joints to become bent and stiff; exercises aim to straighten these joints to the limit and maintain mobility. Home exercise should avoid going beyond the point of pain. A doctor can outline the exercises needed. A Seton Arthro-Pad can be used for knees, elbows, even ankles, and may bring extraordinary relief. They come in three sizes: small, medium and large. They should only be worn for a few days at a time as regular use of supports weakens muscles. Chemists such as Bell & Croydon, Wigmore Street, London, W.1. stock such items.

RHEUMATOID ARTHRITIS affects younger people, more often women. The cause is uncertain although it may be due to a virus. It starts in the small joints of the hands and wrists and may be associated with general ill health. The joints tend to be more hot and angry than in osteoarthritis and may respond to injections of cortisone and cold applications.

During the less acute stages sufferers from both these forms of arthritis may be helped by exercise, massage to surrounding muscles, heat or hydrotherapy. Where active exercise is not possible the physiotherapist may put the joint passively through its full range of movement. This is to prevent stiffness and deformity which can develop rapidly in unused joints. All forms of arthritis can benefit from tablets to reduce inflammation and pain (aspirin, indomethacin, etc.) and rheumatoid arthritics may also be treated by gold injections, penicillamine and cortisone. Some claim benefits from a course of cod liver oil.

Much relief has been brought to sufferers by the modern joint replacement operations.

Pain relief and better mobility, especially in the hip, are achieved in an amazingly short space of time. The main snag in the U.K. is the long N.H.S. waiting lists.

Still's disease, a form of Rheumatoid Arthritis in children, requires treatment in a special centre.

Gout is another form of arthritis (*see* GOUT). There are many other types but the general priorities of management are the same. (*See also* BACKACHE *and* EXERCISE, *page 13*.)

Artificial Insemination. (*See* INFERTILITY)

Artificial Respiration.
Needed when the patient has stopped breathing for himself.

In this emergency NO TIME CAN BE WASTED. Resuscitation must begin AT ONCE with no moments spared to place the patient's (or rescuer's) body comfortably. A drowned person, for instance, must receive artificial respiration as soon as his head is free from the water.

DELAY OF ONE OR TWO SECONDS MAY PROVE FATAL.

At the most, if the first-aider suspects that the patient's throat is badly blocked by false teeth, mud or weeds for instance – he may try to clear this by turning the head to one side and, with one quick, thorough scoop of his finger, sweeping the back of the mouth.

Once artificial respiration has been given for two or three minutes with air coming freely in and out of the lungs, then, and only then, may attention be paid to other details of positioning the patient, of covering him, seeking additional help and so on. But all the time the rescuer must continue to give artificial respiration and keep careful watch.

Method used: **Mouth-to-mouth** (*or mouth-to-nose*).

1. The rescuer breathes air from his own lungs into the patient's lungs, through the patient's mouth or nose. Even though this is air breathed out by the rescuer it still holds enough oxygen for the purpose.

2. THE HEAD MUST BE HELD TILTED WELL BACK WITH THE LOWER JAW PUSHED FORWARD.

When a healthy conscious person is breathing there is plenty of space for the air to move from the mouth and nose to the windpipe (as in picture A). With an unconscious patient lying on his back the tongue is likely to fall backwards, blocking the space between the mouth and the windpipe. Air cannot get through, as in picture B.

Therefore the patient's head is pressed back, so that the nostrils look directly upwards. His lower jaw is *pushed forward* so that the chin juts out, then the tongue moves forward with the lower jaw and the air passages are opened, as in picture C, below.

C.

3. Pinch the nostrils shut with the fingers of one hand and keep the head right back.
4. With the fingers and the thumb of the other hand press the lower jaw forward so that the chin juts out. At the same time get the mouth open. Maintain in this position all the time, as shown in picture D.

D.

5. Take a deep breath.
6. Open your mouth wide. Seal your lips round the patient's open mouth.
7. Blow firmly, but gently, into the patient's mouth and so into his lungs, as shown in picture E.
8. Lift your mouth off, turning your head to look at the patient's chest. If you have been successful

E.

you will see that it has risen and is now falling as the air comes out. Otherwise check for obstruction in the throat. *The above may seem an intricate series of steps. It is not. With practice it can be done as one move which immediately gives air to the patient.*

9. Repeat 5, 6, 7 and 8 for four full, quick breaths. This will load the patient's blood with oxygen. His colour should improve.

10. Now continue at a steady deliberate rate, watching the rise of the chest as guarantee that air is entering the lungs and blowing in again as soon as the chest as fallen.

For children the above would be carried out at a somewhat faster rate, but more gently, depending on the size of the child.

Important safeguards in the mouth-to-mouth method:
(The numbers in brackets refer to the step numbers above)
(3) Pinch the nostrils (not the bony bridge or the extreme tip of the nose).
(4) (a) Get the head back far enough. You should be able to look vertically down on the now closed nostrils.

(b) Keep your fingers away from the patient's lips so that your own lips can form a perfect seal.
(6) Open your mouth widely enough so that it makes a complete seal round the patient's mouth.
(7) Blow from your chest, and not from your cheeks.

(b) Blow only hard enough to make the patient's chest rise.
(8) If the chest has not moved, check that you have the patient's nose closed and that you are keeping his head far enough back.
(10) Blow steadily after the first four quick breaths. If you continue too rapidly you will tire yourself and may even feel faint.

(*See* ASPHYXIA.)

The Publishers are indebted to the Red Cross for the information on which the above is based.

Artificial Teeth. (*See* DENTURES)

Asphyxia. (*See* ARTIFICIAL RESPIRATION *on page 35.*)

This is the condition of suffocation in which the body is deprived of air, or more specifically of oxygen (*see* ANAEMIA). Asphyxia may arise in several ways. The air passages may be blocked as in strangulation when the windpipe is compressed, or in young children who sometimes get food or other objects stuck in the back of the throat. It may be produced by breathing gases which lack oxygen, as in a smoke filled house during a blazing fire. It may result from electric shock, when the muscles which move the chest and draw air into the lungs become paralysed, or it may arise in drowning when water enters the lungs. Whatever the cause, normal breathing must be started as soon as possible to prevent death.

If a young child chokes and goes blue in the face with something stuck in the throat he should be picked up by the legs, held upside down, and thumped vigorously on the back to dislodge the block. Medical aid should be summoned urgently, and if the above does not free the air passage, a finger should be pushed as far down the throat as possible in an attempt to free the obstruction. If this fails, a sharp blow just below the breastbone will sometimes clear it.

If after poisoning by fumes or coal gas, electric shock, or drowning, breathing does not start immediately, ARTIFICIAL RESPIRATION must be given without delay.

Asthma.

Asthma is a condition of periodic and reversible constriction of the breathing tubes and results in wheezy and difficult breathing. It is often hereditary and due to abnormal sensitivity to substances in the environment. (*See* ALLERGY.)

Wheezy bronchitis in babies is not necessarily the same; it responds well to treatment and many children grow out of it.

Patients with asthma should be investigated in an attempt to identify their particular sensitivities. The commonest substances causing asthma are house dust mite and animal fur. The patient may be greatly helped by avoiding the relevant animals; the bedroom, including bed and bedcovers, should be vacuum cleaned daily and bedding should be of synthetic material. The bedroom should be sparsely furnished and clothes kept elsewhere. Mattresses are a major source of house dust and should be sealed in plastic bags. (The house dust mite is a tiny "insect" invisible to the naked eye.)

Desensitisation to house dust mite by the use of a course of injections may reduce asthma attacks in some cases. Many medicines (tablets and inhalers to open up the breathing tubes, Intal and cortisone both as tablets and inhaler) are available to prevent and control attacks. When a severe attack does not improve rapidly on the usual prescribed medicine a doctor must be called as more urgent treatment may be needed (injections, oxygen, etc.). Do not over-use your inhaler in a misguided attempt to avoid troubling your doctor. Failure to gain relief may mean that you need urgent medical reassessment.

Moderate exercise and special breathing exercises may help some. Asthma can, however, be made worse by exercise and some sufferers may need to use Intal inhalers before playing games, running, etc. Swimming is a particularly useful activity for asthmatics as it is less likely to provoke breathing constriction and can be used in a graduated training programme which your doctor may outline.

Athlete's Foot.

Itchy fungus infection of the skin between the toes; common among the young who take part in swimming and barefoot activities. Avoid public baths and showers till the condition has cleared. Mycota, Mycil, or Canesten cream and powders usually cure but must be continued for two weeks after apparent cure. (*See* TINEA.)

Autism.

A distressing form of mental illness in young children. The child is emotionally unresponsive and fails to relate to family and surroundings. This may or may not be associated with other forms of delay in development. Urgent psychiatric treatment is required.

B

Baby Feeding. (*See* INFANT FEEDING)

Backache.

A common complaint, usually due to a type of muscular rheumatism, or may follow an unaccustomed strain. A hot bath followed by a rub over the affected part with linament will often cure. Overweight, bad posture, and occupations involving much lifting, standing or bending tend to cause backache. Mental stress is also an important cause.

Severe immobilizing backache of sudden onset and pain down the leg(s) suggests a slipped disc (*see* SLIPPED DISC) requiring urgent medical advice.

Those with a tendency to recurrent pain should have a hard mattress and put supporting boards under it during acute attacks. Weight loss and attention to general fitness help where appropriate. Exercise during pain-free spells helps to strengthen the muscles in the small of the back. These include lying prone (face downwards) and raising head and shoulders from the ground ten times, followed by raising the legs similarly ten times night and morning.

A supporting corset eases pain but should be reserved for acute episodes as muscles become weak if always supported. In women a chronic low backache is occasionally due to disease or displacement of the womb and in both sexes persistent backache can be a symptom of some internal disorder. If it persists more than a week or two see a doctor, but the majority are not serious and disappear with simple treatment and time. Orthodox investigations of backache often reveal no obvious cause and sufferers are frequently dissatisfied with treatment. Pressure from patients has resulted in various backache groups being formed in the U.K. and it will be interesting to see if more precise treatment and diagnosis will be forthcoming. (*See* ARTHRITIS, EXERCISE, *page 13, and* OSTEOARTHRITIS.)

Bad Breath. (*See* HALITOSIS)

Balanitis.
Inflammation due to infection under the foreskin in boys and men. After the age of four the foreskin should be fully retracted daily for purposes of washing. In this way the problem should be avoided. (*See* CIRCUMCISION *and* PHIMOSIS.)

Baldness.
Loss of hair. Ordinary baldness is almost entirely confined to men and often runs in families. There is no cure as

lost hair cannot re-grow. Hair tonics are useless. Where there is a family history it may be worth trying to prevent hair loss by scalp care. Avoid tight hats. The hair should be washed with a good shampoo weekly. Rinse out with warm, then cold water. On the day following the hair should be left alone, but on other days of the week five minutes' massage to the scalp should be carried out night and morning. The diet should be rich in protein, calcium and all the vitamins, particularly B and C. (Inexpensive Becosym vitamin tablets have been found helpful by some people – including doctors).

Female hormones have been found to be useful in the treatment of hair loss in women.

If in spite of scalp care, ordinary (male) baldness ensues there is no effective treatment other than the use of wigs, toupees or expensive surgery. It may console the sufferer to think of baldness as an extreme form of the normal masculine hair pattern of recession at the temples.

Total loss of all scalp and body hair (*Alopecia Totalis*) is an unusual condition occurring in both sexes. In the U.K., wigs may be supplied by the N.H.S. in cases of total alopecia or where baldness is causing serious mental suffering.

"Hair transplants" can be obtained in a few private clinics. Patches of hair-bearing skin from the back of the neck are transferred to the head – a few at a time – so the procedure is time-consuming as well as costly. But it usually works.

Another type affecting both sexes is *Alopecia Areata* where hair falls out in patches. This may follow a serious illness, or a lot of worry. In this type of baldness lost hair grows again although this may take months. The process may be speeded by cortisone applications and treatment for any anxiety.

Bartholin's Glands.

Tiny glands on either side of the vaginal opening, they may become infected or blocked to form a cyst. Treatment is by a minor operation.

Bed Wetting. (*See* ENURESIS, INCONTINENCE, *etc.*)

Bee Stings. (*See* STINGS)

Bell's Palsy.
Paralysis of one half of the face probably due to a virus infection of the nerve which supplies the face muscles. The face is twisted away from the affected side. Injection of a substance (A.C.T.H.) which produces cortisone may speed recovery but even without treatment the condition usually clears completely in weeks.

Bends.
Occurs in divers who have surfaced too quickly. As pressure is rapidly reduced, gases bubble out of the blood causing limb and abdominal pains. Treatment is recompression in a special chamber.

Bile.
Greenish yellow liquid made by the liver and poured into the intestines via the bile duct. It aids digestion in many ways. (*See* GALL BLADDER.)

Biliousness.
A lay term describing a temporary digestive upset, particularly nausea and vomiting. *Consult* ACIDOSIS *and* DYSPEPSIA.

Biopsy.
Removal of a small piece of tissue for laboratory examination.

Birth.
Normally the baby is expelled from the mother's body at about the end of the 40th week of pregnancy. Labour is divided into three stages. The first consists of a dilatation of the neck of the womb, when the regular contractions or "pains" gradually enlarge the opening until it is big enough for baby to pass through. The second stage is the gradual descent of the baby from the womb through the female passage (vagina) until it leaves the mother's body. In the third stage the womb contracts in size and finally expels the placenta, or afterbirth. This is a large mass of tissue

attached to the inside of the womb from which the baby draws nourishment from the mother.

Normally the patient should be under the care of a doctor or midwife. It sometimes happens that a birth occurs in some out-of-the-way place or starts early and unexpectedly before medical aid can be summoned. Under these circumstances a lay person may have to help the mother. Labour is usually heralded by a show of mucus (slime) and blood or sometimes by "the waters" breaking. Successive labours tend to be shorter by several hours and anyone with a history of a previously rapid labour should make allowances for this. If the previous birth was extremely quick it is often wisest for an arrangement to be made whereby the mother is taken into hospital a week or so early.

When the contraction pains last more than half a minute and occur at regular intervals of fifteen to twenty minutes it means that the first stage of labour is under way. At this point (or if the waters break) the patient is advised to enter hospital or contact the doctor. If this help is delayed a warm bedroom should be prepared and the bed made with freshly laundered linen. The mother may lie on her side or back. At the end of the first stage, contractions occur roughly every three minutes or so and last for about one and a half minutes. When the second stage begins the mother usually has a strong desire to bear down and can be encouraged to do so. When the baby's head appears it should be restrained for a little by pressure from the well-washed hand of the person helping. At this point the mother should be asked to pant and not push. This is to prevent *sudden* stretching of the external parts which might get torn.

After the head is born the rest of the body normally follows quickly and easily. The baby will still be attached to the mother by the umbilical cord, and this should be tied in two places, an inch or two apart, with clean thread six inches away from the baby. It should then be cut *between the threads* with clean (preferably boiled) scissors, which will prevent bleeding from the cord. There is no hurry about this cord cutting: if suitable implements are not available the afterbirth can be delivered whilst still attached to the cord; indeed leave well alone if medical help is expected within an hour or less. The important thing is to check on the condition of the baby and mother. If bleeding is excessive treat as below. *If no medical help is forthcoming that day* and the above implements are not to hand the cord can be tied with fine clean string and cut with a clean sharp knife (even teeth in emergency). The baby may be smacked once or twice if he does not breathe or cry within twenty seconds of the birth and then should be wrapped in warm clothing and left in peace. If there is no response to smacking, *gentle* mouth to mouth breathing should be used until medical help arrives (*see* ARTIFICIAL RESPIRATION). Mucus may be cleared from the baby's nose and mouth by suction through any available tubing or drinking straw.

The mother should be covered in warm bedclothes, and she will probably produce the "afterbirth" in a short while. If the afterbirth is not delivered within an hour or so the patient is in danger from excessive bleeding. If there *is* considerable bleeding after the baby is born raise the foot of the bed (e.g. on a chair) so that the mother's head is lower than her buttocks. She should be kept especially warm. In the event of such haemorrhage, *in remote areas where medical help is not available*, firm downwards pressure of the hand on the stomach above the uterus (felt as a firm muscular swelling just below the navel) should expel the afterbirth. If bleeding continues, the uterus (womb) can be squeezed firmly by a hand placed on the abdomen above, when usually the womb will contract to stop the blood loss. The afterbirth should be saved for the doctor's inspection so that he may see if it is complete. *No unqualified person should attempt to conduct a birth unless there is no alternative, and every effort must be made to get a doctor, midwife or nurse at the earliest*. Apart from haemorrhage the birth outlined above is a normal one. *It must be again stressed births can go wrong very suddenly and it would be a very grave matter if every attempt had not been made to get medical aid quickly*.

More complicated births such as breech deliveries (buttocks first) and forceps deliveries can occur, which are outside our scope. Under modern conditions the mother experiences very little more discomfort than with a normal birth (local or general anaesthetic may be used) and the assisted delivery may be life saving.

Natural Childbirth.

It is no longer felt that natural childbirth can be completely painless, and any mother who feels the need for pain relief should request this. Knowledge about pregnancy and labour and some form of relaxation exercises help the woman to cope with labour and need the minimum amount of painkillers and sedatives. *In the normal birth, the less afraid the woman is, the less will be her pain.*

Grantly Dick-Read was one of the pioneers of natural childbirth who thought that by overcoming fear and by reducing ignorance with knowledge, women could have a "natural", relatively painless birth. Many modifications of his ideas followed. At present in the U.K. most women are taught a modified version of psychoprophylaxis plus general relaxation. The aim is to "distract" the woman from the pain of the contractions by training her to *concentrate* on tightening other muscles or performing breathing exercises. This together with the support of her husband who can be a useful companion during the first stage, can lead to a comfortable labour. It does not guarantee a *normal* labour; complications may still arise and the mother should not feel that this is due to any failure on her part. The National Childbirth Trust advises women on all matters relating to pregnancy, psychoprophylaxis and birth.

At the other end of the spectrum from childbirth with the minimum of drugs is a trend towards epidural anaesthesia (*see* ANAESTHETICS). Ideally, the mother can spend the whole labour free of pain. Here, the forceps delivery percentage tends to be rather high as there is little urge to push in the second stage.

Caesarian Operation.

The operation by which a living child is taken from the mother's womb by an incision through the abdomen. The name is derived from Roman times. Caesarian section is not particularly difficult and can be used in cases where normal birth might be hazardous. It should have no serious after-effects, and many patients consider it less unpleasant than normal labour. A Caesarian section is no bar to having subsequent children. The scar can usually be hidden by a bikini! After a Caesarian the mother takes a little longer to find her feet but all the advice below applies.

All mothers are apt to feel low a few days after delivery – "fourth day blues". This should disappear a week or so later, and a mother feeling seriously depressed after the first ten days should see the doctor urgently as post-natal depression can be severe, but responds well to prompt treatment.

There is a lot of tiredness in the early weeks after a baby, as demands are great and sleep disturbed. Mothers should take as much rest as possible between the demands of the infant and take advantage (without guilt) of offers of help from fond relatives or friends. Apart from establishing a routine for the baby, this is not the time to get obsessional about housework. Aim to get out with your husband at least once a week!

Mothers should take extra iron for a year after delivery to replenish iron stores. They should be sure to attend for post-natal examination six weeks after delivery to check that all is well and for contraceptive advice.

Birth Control. (*See* CONTRACEPTION)

Birthmark. (*Naevus*)

There are several types of mark which may be apparent on the skin at birth. The "port wine" stain varies from pink to dark bluish red and unfortunately often occurs on the face. Treatment is by the application of liquid nitrogen and more recently by laser (intensely focussed light beams) therapy. Results, however, are rather disappointing and cosmetic covering cream is often necessary. There are however some excellent creams such as "Covermark" and "Keromask" which can be bought or obtained on doctor's prescription in severe cases.

The "strawberry mark" is quite a common naevus. It may be inconspicuous at birth and then to the distress of the baby's parents, often grows alarmingly in size and thickness in the early months, becoming purple in colour. In spite of this the outlook is excellent as after growing for perhaps as long as two or three years it normally shrinks to form a white flat patch by the age of four to seven. Often no treatment is needed but if necessary the flat patch can be removed after full shrinkage has occurred. Surgery in the early stages, when the mark is large and full of blood vessels, would be risky and leave an unnecessarily large scar. Parents can be reassured that a strawberry mark or "cavernous haemangioma" will always get smaller in the long run. They should not think they are being fobbed off by a busy doctor when he reassures them on this. The only indication for operation earlier is when there is recurrent bleeding due to friction from clothing, etc.

The tiny pale pink marks on the eyelids and back of the neck in about 50% of babies fade naturally and are nothing to worry about.

Blackheads. (*See* ACNE)

Small black spots in the skin due to a collection of debris in the openings of the oil producing glands. The general treatment for ACNE and blackheads is the same, and the two conditions are commonly found together. Individual blackheads can sometimes be removed by soaking well in hot water and pressing with the end of a key which has a hole in the end (e.g. small clock key). Firm pressure with the end of the key around the blackhead will often cause it to pop out.

Bleeding. (*See* HAEMORRHAGE *and* BIRTH)

Blood Groups.

Blood can be divided into four main groups – A, B, O and AB. These depend on the presence or absence of anti-bodies which will attack and break down the red cells of a different group, e.g. if blood group A is given to a patient of group O – the antibodies of the patient destroy the trans-fused red cells causing severe illness with shaking and fever.

The A, B, O groups can be further sub-divided into rhesus positive and rhesus negative (*see* RHESUS FACTOR). All patients must receive the correct ABO and rhesus group blood for successful transfusion.

Patients often wish to know their blood group. The best

way to find out is to enrol as a blood donor. You will be tested immediately. In disputed paternity, blood groups can sometimes be used to prove that a man is *not* the father; they can never prove that *he is*.

Blood Pressure.

The heart is a specially adapted muscle which pumps blood through blood vessels around the body. This results in the blood being under pressure, and since the vessels become hardened with age, and have less "give", the blood pressure tends to rise. It is thus *normal* to have a rather higher blood pressure at sixty than at twenty. At an earlier age in certain conditions, kidney disease, gland disease, and sometimes for no apparent reason, the pressure may rise to dangerous levels. The chief risks are that the heart may be unable to cope or a blood vessel may burst in some organ such as the brain (*see* STROKE).

Even in normal persons the pressure varies greatly and there is a wide margin of increased pressure that the heart and vessels can deal with without great danger. Lay people tend to be frightened of hypertension, but those with a moderate rise in the pressure may live for years. I have known sufferers who reached great age, and died from something unconnected. Be advised by your doctor. He will probably arrange tests to see if there is a curable cause and check for any sign of adverse effect on heart or kidneys. He will suggest a reducing diet if you are overweight, abstention from smoking and reduction of animal fats if these are indicated. He may perhaps prescribe tablets to reduce the pressure such as diuretics (water eliminating tablets) methyldopa or betablockers. There may be no symptoms of blood pressure; it is often found during a routine medical insurance examination. Occasionally headaches and giddiness are found to be caused by raised blood pressure. Once you are known to have raised blood pressure you will need the pressure checked occasionally, (be guided by your own doctor), as treatment may need to be adjusted. You should continue accustomed activities but if you have taken no exercise for years do not suddenly take up squash; start gradually with short walks and build up.

Blood Tests.

Many conditions can be checked on by blood tests. Anaemia and other blood diseases can be detected as can kidney and liver disorders and some venereal diseases. Too much cholesterol (a fatty substance associated with heart and artery disease) may be found and many chronic illnesses, glandular diseases and forms of arthritis can be confirmed by blood tests. The blood levels of alcohol, drugs and poisons may be measured (it is sometimes useful to know if the patient is taking his tablets!) One value of tests is that, if negative, they reassure the patient who may be fearing the worst. (*See* BLOOD GROUPS.)

Blood Transfusion.

This technique of transferring blood from a healthy donor to a patient saves many lives. Operations, once impossible, can be performed with relative safety, and accident cases, perhaps bleeding after childbirth, have a better chance of recovery, as have some kinds of anaemia; "Blood banks" are kept to be readily available in emergency, and giving blood for transfusion is safe, and simple. Everyone who can should volunteer. (*See* BLOOD GROUPS.)

Blue Baby.

Person born with heart defects hindering the blood being pumped efficiently to the lungs. This results in blood lacking oxygen being sent to the rest of the body so that the patient looks blue or dusky. Good results are now obtained by surgery and one of my patients with this history has had her own normal baby after an uncomplicated pregnancy and birth.

Boils.

Abscesses develop in the skin due to infection by germs. These usually enter through small openings of the sweat glands. The best home remedy is to apply Anaflex powder spray and cover with a non-stick (Melolin) dressing. Do not squeeze. If it does not clear or if boils appear in crops, consult your doctor as penicillin should put matters right. Attention to cleanliness particularly of the hands plus a balanced diet should keep boils to a minimum. A sufferer should keep to his own towels and facecloths which should be boiled after use. Disposable tissues and towels are even safer. (*See* ABSCESS.)

Bone Infection. (*See* OSTEOMYELITIS)

Brain and Body Scanners. (*Scan*)

A recent British invention using computer assisted X-rays to scan the brain and the rest of the body. The resulting pictures show details of structures deep in the brain or body and can help detect many diseases *early*.

Breast.

A normally inactive gland which after a birth begins to function and produce milk (lactation). Sometimes perseverance is needed before breast feeding is established, and a mother should try because breast milk is best for the infant. It contains valuable substances for warding off infection which cannot be replaced artificially. *Where there is a family history of allergy (asthma and eczema), breast feeding may protect the baby against later allergic illness*. It should be continued for as long as possible, perhaps up to nine months although of course other solids may be introduced at four to six months. Mothers who breast feed have a lower incidence of breast tumours developing later. Sometimes during lactation germs enter the breast, which becomes painful and inflamed, and a breast abscess (*see* ABSCESS) may develop. This is usually preceded by a sore, cracked nipple; modern sprays and careful drying after washing with plain water should prevent this condition but if it does occur seek medical advice at the onset so that abscess formation is prevented. Antibiotics can cure at this stage and breast feeding continues. If an abscess does develop hot poultices may be applied as an emergency but urgent medical advice is required.

Any lump in the breast, or problem, at any age, calls for medical advice.

Self examination of the breasts

Examine your breasts regularly, at the same time each month, e.g. the day after your period ceases. If you have passed the *"change of life"*, the first day of the calendar month.

Examine the upper part of the breast, including the armpit, then the lower and central parts of the breast.

With your right hand, examine the whole of your left breast, as shown in the diagrams, starting at the armpit. Then examine the right breast with the left hand. Follow the sequence shown in Fig. 3, nos. 1 to 4.

FIG.3 Self examination of the breasts

It is important to use the flat of your hand, keeping your finger tips held lightly together, making sure that the finger tips, the most sensitive part of the hand, follow the same path as the flat of your hand.

Should you find a lump in the breast, or any of the following "warning signs", which was not present last month, go to your doctor and say "I have a lump in my breast" or "There is something wrong which I was not aware of last month".

Tell him carefully what difference you have noticed, and ask his advice. Through lack of knowledge some women only report to their doctor when a lump or swelling in the breast has been present a long time. The following points may be "warning signs" that something could be wrong:

1. A lump or swelling in the breast.
2. Pain in the breast, not confined to the time just before a period.
3. A stained discharge from the nipple, or skin trouble around the nipple, or a "pulling in" of the nipple.
4. An alteration in the appearance of the breast, e.g. dimpling or puckering of the skin.
5. A change in shape or size of one breast, compared with the other breast, which has occurred during the month.

Most of the above symptoms require specialist investigation. Tests include special X-rays and drawing off fluid if it is a cystic swelling. If there is a doubt, the specialist will wish to remove the lump. Often the lump is removed and the test is reported as satisfactory. If laboratory testing done during the operation shows that the lump is malignant the surgeon will usually go ahead with mastectomy (removal of breast). This is always explained to you in advance.

The operation of mastectomy is not very serious although the psychological blow is immense. The Mastectomy Association of Croydon, London, formed by women who have had this operation, gives general advice and support.

The patient is fitted with an artificial breast and special bra as soon as possible and again the Mastectomy Association can often help with any problems.

Radiotherapy and drugs may be given after operation if your specialist feels this necessary. Careful follow-up is needed and the patient should never lose touch with her specialist unless discharged. The outlook can be good if the lump is caught early. I know several sprightly eighty year olds who had successful operations thirty years ago.

Information on self-examination of the breasts courtesy of South-West Thames Regional Cancer Services.

Bronchiectasis.

A chronic lung infection due to weakness and distortion of the smaller breathing tubes or bronchi. It can sometimes be helped by an operation to remove the affected part of the lung. It can be an after-effect of whooping cough and is one good reason for having infants immunized in the first year of life.

Bronchiolitis.

A severe infection of the smallest breathing tubes in babies. Any baby with breathing difficulty needs urgent medical attention. A humid warm atmosphere helps temporarily. (*See* CROUP.)

Bronchitis.

A common complaint, especially in winter, and often follows a "cold". Smokers and workers in dusty, polluted atmospheres are most affected. In babies bronchitis can be a short, easily cured illness: in adults chronic bronchitis tends to be a recurrent problem.

It may not at first be noticeable except for a morning cough, but after the additional insult of a virus infection the lining of the breathing tubes becomes swollen and inflamed. There is often pain in the chest, raised temperature, cough, and the production of sputum. The patient is best in bed in a warm atmosphere, and a cough mixture such as Benylin may help. Lemon and honey mixtures are soothing and if there is fever Disprin or paracetamol are indicated. Inhalation of Friars' Balsam is a well tried remedy but medical advice is needed as antibiotics may be required. Stop smoking for good, as this illness tends to recur if the bronchi are repeatedly irritated. The end result of repeated attacks can be extreme shortness of breath even at rest, and this must be avoided. (*See* SMOKING.)

Apart from stopping smoking ask your doctor's advice about anti-flu injections in the autumn and let him know when you have a minor cold. He may wish you to start antibiotics at the first sign. (This does not apply to the vast majority of "healthy" folk who should rarely need antibiotics.) Stay in bed with bronchitis since there is a danger of pneumonia. Keep your legs moving while on bedrest. Do not go outdoors till fit.

Broncho-pneumonia.

A type of pneumonia in which the infection spreads from the breathing tubes, or bronchi, into the lung substance. (*See* PNEUMONIA.)

Bronchoscopy.

A procedure whereby the specialist uses an illuminated tube to look down the large breathing tubes and by which he can detect certain illnesses and take samples for testing.

Brucellosis.

Infection caught by contact with infected cattle or their milk and characterised by intermittent fever, aches and pains. As symptoms are vague it is difficult to diagnose and should be considered whenever there is unexplained, persistent fever. People in rural areas should avoid drinking unpasteurised milk. Frequent veterinary inspection and testing of cattle is important for the prevention of this distressing disease.

Bruises.

Caused by violence which does not break the skin, but injures the tissues. Colour changes are due to bleeding into the damaged tissues. The only treatment is time, which brings a return to normal. If painful a cold compress – lint wrung out in ice-cold water – helps. A black eye is one variety of bruise. The proverbial beef steak is no use. In children a loving cuddle is often the best medicine.

Bunion. (*See* BURSA)

Burns.

Injury caused by excessive heat to part of the body so as to damage or kill the tissues. It may be due to a flame, a hot object, excessive sunlight, or boiling water when the condition is called a SCALD. There is no practical difference between a burn and scald. Burns may also be caused by chemicals. In mild cases there may be only reddening of the skin (first degree). In second degree there is blistering and in third degree, the whole skin thickness, is destroyed, and the area appears charred. There are two chief dangers. First is *shock*, a severe form of collapse which follows extensive burns. Second is infection. When the tissues are killed or injured they cannot defend against invasion by germs, so that burns easily become infected and "fester". The *immediate* home treatment of burns (dry or wet) is to cool in cold running water; damage and pain can thus be reduced. Continue cooling until there is no further pain (up to thirty minutes if necessary). If the burn is severe or large (e.g. a blistered area more than 1″ (25 mm) across in a child or 3″ (75 mm) in an adult) shock should be treated by wrapping unburned areas with extra clothing or a blanket and giving a warm, sugared drink if patient is conscious. Urgent medical treatment is required for large burns but *initial cooling is always necessary*. Smaller burns can be covered by any antiseptic cream and a freshly laundered handkerchief. Later they can be dressed with acriflex cream or betadine spray and covered with a non-stick melo-lin dressing. If "festering" occurs consult your doctor who may give antibiotics.

Bursa. (*Bursitis*)

A small sac containing fluid which protects part of the body from injury. It is usually found over some prominent bone which it cushions. If a bursa becomes inflamed it is known as *bursitis*. This most commonly occurs in the feet, elbows and knees. There is a small bursa at the base of each of the big toes on the inner side. This commonly becomes inflamed through wearing too tight shoes and is often known as a BUNION. If protected from pressure by wearing loose shoes or slippers, it will often subside. A small pad round the bunion may help. Where symptoms ascribed to bunions are in fact due to rigidity of the toe joints (*hallux rigidus*) foot exercises such as picking up marbles or bean bags with the toes may help.

In a true bunion the bursa may become infected and discharge pus. The treatment is rest, heat and antibiotics. An operation may be the best way of preventing further trouble. Final results are usually good although a long convalescence with several weeks hobbling on crutches will have to be endured. Bunions are agony; worse than toothache and those who wear tight shoes will probably pay a painful price. Every child should be allowed enough room for the foot to grow within the shoe. Parents must keep a watchful eye to see that the toes do not become cramped.

In the knee there is a bursa over the knee-cap which may become inflamed if much kneeling is done (housemaid's knee). This subsides with rest, and it may be necessary to avoid kneeling. Exercising the parts, but not to the extent of agony, can help to dissipate adhesions and prevent recurrence. A knee or elbow arthro-pad worn for a day or two (not regularly because of weakening effect on muscles) may help. This should be obtainable at good chemists.

C

Caesarian Section. (*See* BIRTH)

Calculus.

The medical term for "stone". Stones may form in organs such as the gall bladder, kidneys or the urinary bladder, and cause pain and other disturbances. Once a stone has formed and causes trouble, removal by an operation is generally necessary. Drugs are now available which dissolve gall stones but recurrence after stopping treatment may be a problem. (*See* GALL BLADDER, KIDNEY DISEASE *and* STONES.)

Cancer.

This condition is all too common, and is the third most frequent cause of death. The term "cancer" covers a group of allied disorders which have in common the unrestrained growth of some small part of the body with the formation of a lump or tumour. Normally the growth of any particular part of the body is carefully regulated to meet with its requirements. When some part is injured the cells (minute living structures) of which it is composed multiply until the injury is made good, but the whole process is controlled. In the condition of cancer, for some reason, a group of cells starts to multiply abnormally and continues to do so, disorganising the normal working of the body. Sometimes groups of these cells may be carried to distant parts of the body by the blood and there set up fresh tumours. If the process continues unchecked some vital organ will eventually become so disorganised that life cannot continue. It is vital *the lay person should not take the all-too-common view that cancer is incurable. In many cases it is curable if taken early – that is the point.* The most effective treatment, in numerous instances, is still surgery, which means cutting out the affected part.

If all the cancer cells are removed the condition will be cured. The smaller the tumour, the less chance it has had to spread, and the more likely is complete cure.

There are also other valuable means of treatment such as radiotherapy, anti-tumour drugs, certain hormones and cortisone. Research indicates that eight out of ten cancers are due to chemicals in the environment. Perhaps the greatest hope is prevention. Methods for detecting and identifying cancer-producing chemicals are being developed and will help to clean up our surroundings. Sources are industrial waste, car exhausts and cigarette smoke.

New treatments being developed include high energy irradiation such as neutron beams. New drugs and new combinations of old drugs are showing promise in some cancers.

The illness is not common before 40 and the incidence increases with age. Perhaps the cells become less efficient at dealing with injury due to irritants over this age. **THE KEYNOTE OF SUCCESS IS EARLY TREATMENT.** Anyone who has a symptom which does not go inside a few weeks should consult a doctor. Danger signals are a lump in breast (*see* BREAST) or testicle, etc., persistent cough (more than three weeks), persistent change in bowel habit, loss of weight, persistent or recurrent pain and the appearance of blood, for example from the bowels, in urine, from the mouth after coughing or vomiting, from the nipple or from the vagina after the menopause or between periods. The chances are there may be some other explanation which your doctor will be able to put right. If your doctor is suspicious he will be able to advise tests to establish the diagnosis. (*See* LEUKAEMIA *and* CERVIX.)

Car Sickness. (*See* TRAVEL SICKNESS.)

Carbuncle.
Similar to a boil but the infection is deeper. A boil discharges through one opening; a carbuncle may have several. For a small carbuncle the treatment is similar *(see* BOIL) but for most consult a doctor. Antibiotics can cure.

Cardiac.   Pertaining to the heart. (*See* HEART DISEASE.)

Cartilage.
A pad of "gristle" in many joints which acts as a buffer between bones. The common one to cause trouble is in the knee. A twist may cause it to tear with acute pain in the knee which often becomes locked and swollen. Sometimes the symptoms may subside with rest, but often it is necessary to remove the cartilage by a simple operation to save further trouble. It may be worth wearing a knee support pad for a few days while trying the resting cure.

Cataract.
A condition, usually occurring in older people, in which the lens of the eye becomes clouded, (*see* Fig. 7, *page 96*), so that less light reaches the retina. Vision becomes progressively worse but the outlook is good. Sometimes the condition becomes arrested, or affects one eye only, and in any case it is possible to operate and remove the opacity. Thick glasses must be worn after the operation to focus the light.

Catarrh.
A rather vague term but usually taken to mean a stuffed-up feeling in head and nose, with or without nasal discharge and is sometimes associated with a feeling of sticky fluid dripping down the back of the throat. These symptoms are normal in the week or two following a cold or flu. Children tend to have twice as many colds as adults and

thus in winter may seem to have persistent snuffles and catarrh. A constant running nose and mouth-breathing in a child may indicate large adenoids. Many "catarrhal" children however out-grow the condition at about seven years as their nasal passages enlarge and become less easily blocked. A foul nasal discharge in a child suggests a foreign body e.g. a bead, stuck in the nose.

The catarrh which follows a cold can be relieved by inhaling the vapour of Friars' Balsam (one teaspoonful to a pint of boiling water). If catarrh persists for more than three weeks after a cold there may be underlying sinusitis which can be treated by your doctor. (*See* ANTRUM.)

Allergy such as hay fever causes watery catarrh, frequent sneezing and "stuffed-up" nose. Allergic subjects tend to develop nasal polyps (thickened folds of the lining of the nose) which increase the catarrh. The piece of cartilage which divides the nasal passages is deviated to one side in some people. Stuffiness and blockage can then occur on the narrow side. This can be helped by a minor operation.

Other causes of catarrh include *smoking,* a polluted or damp atmosphere and *excessive use of decongestant nose drops.*

Catheter.
A tube for withdrawing fluid from a cavity – e.g. the bladder.

Cellulitis.
A spreading skin infection due to a germ. The area affected becomes red, swollen and painful, and the patient usually has fever. Get expert treatment, for nowadays it is usually rapidly curable.

Cerebral.
Pertaining to the brain. (*See* STROKE.)

Cervical Spondylosis.
Osteoarthritis occurring in the neck joints. Symptoms may include aching and stiffness in the neck as well as pain, weakness and "pins and needles" in the arms when the nerves emerging through canals in the vertebrae in the neck

become irritated by pressure from swollen joints. A collar of foam or plastic worn for one to three months will usually bring relief as may exercise, traction and radiant heat. (*See* ARTHRITIS *and* OSTEOARTHRITIS.)

Cervix.

The neck of the womb which opens in childbirth. Cancer of the cervix is a common but, hopefully, preventable form of cancer in women and can occur at a relatively young age. An easy test (cervical smear) is useful in detecting early changes. The procedure takes seconds and is no more uncomfortable than an internal examination. The smear is examined in a laboratory and altered cells can be spotted before they have invaded other tissues (i.e. become malignant).

Early disease can be treated by removing part of the cervix (coning). In other cases hysterectomy (removal of the womb) is performed and the patient is carefully followed up.

Extreme care in hygiene of the penis and underside of the foreskin is vital as it is thought the "debris" which collects may contribute to cervical cancer. (*See also* BIRTH, CONTRACEPTION, INFERTILITY *and* UTERUS.)

Chancre. (*See* SYPHILIS)

Change of Life. (*See* MENOPAUSE)

Chicken Pox. (*See* SHINGLES)

One of the infective illnesses of childhood, caused by a virus. Most children catch it, usually during school years. A second attack is rare. Incubation is usually about two to three weeks, i.e. it takes that time for symptoms to develop after invasion by the virus. Sometimes the child is off colour before the spots develop, but usually spots are the first symptoms. At first they are small red bumps, but develop a white top containing fluid and later form a crust. The spots usually appear on the chest, and spread to the face, scalp and the upper parts of limbs. The child often has fever, and is best in bed during this stage. The patient should be kept from others who have not had the disease until all the scabs have come off as these may be infective. This usually takes about two weeks. Complications of chicken pox are rare (though it can be worse in adults) and uneventful recovery the rule. The same germ can cause shingles later in life.

Chilblain.

A red, painful itching area on the extremities after exposure to cold. (Most often on feet, hands and nose.) It is usually associated with poor circulation. Those subject to chilblains should take care in cold weather, wearing warm socks and gloves. Extremities should not be warmed suddenly, at the fire or in hot water, after being cold, as this may worsen the condition. Some sufferers are helped by calcium, vitamin D or vitamin K tablets in winter. Vasodilator tablets (which open up the small blood vessels) such as "Pernivit" are helpful if taken regularly after meals in winter. Akrotherm and Pernomol ointments are soothing.

Choking.

Choking on food is common and can be life-threatening. Get behind the victim, place one clenched fist midway between navel and rib cage. Grasp this fist with your other hand, give a sudden firm upward thrust. This thrust should dislodge the food (Heimlich Manoeuvre). Repeat several times if unsuccessful. If alone, do this upward thrust yourself or try a sudden bend over a chairback. If there is distress or breathing difficulty get medical help to prevent chest complications. Children should avoid boiled sweets, nuts, etc. Particles of food, e.g. peanut fragments, can occasionally be inhaled causing breathing difficulties. Children are mostly at risk so get prompt medical advice if alarmed. This could avoid later chest complications.

Cholera.

An infectious disease marked by severe watery diarrhoea which leads to fluid depletion, cramps and collapse. It needs urgent medical care. It is caused by a germ invading the bowels and can be spread by contaminated water supplies. It occurs in epidemics particularly in Asia, Africa and the Mediterranean so it is important for travellers to these and any other risky areas to be inoculated.

Vaccinations provide partial protection; the best prevention is scrupulous care over food and drink (especially drinking water, shellfish and uncooked food).

Cholesterol.

A fatty substance which circulates in the blood. Too much seems to result in premature hardening of the arteries and heart disease. Probably most people would be wise to reduce the intake of animal fat. Vegetable oils are low in cholesterol. (*See* ARTERIOSCLEROSIS *and* HEART DISEASE.)

Chorea.

Popularly known as St. Vitus' Dance. It is now rare in the U.K. It may occur in children and adolescents following a throat infection. (*See* RHEUMATIC FEVER.) Uncontrolled movements occur due to a temporary brain disturbance. Treatment is bed rest during the acute stage and a prolonged course of antibiotics. The outcome is usually good.

Circumcision.

Surgical removal of the male foreskin – practised as a Jewish or other religious rite. In the U.K. it is generally considered unnecessary as most infants have a fully retractable foreskin by six. The foreskin helps to protect the glans-penis from napkin irritation. After this, daily washing beneath the foreskin should prevent inflammation or infection. If the foreskin opening appears to be pinhole size, or ballooning occurs when water is passed or there are repeated attacks of balanitis – circumcision may be necessary on medical grounds. Do not attempt to pull back the foreskin before three or four years. It is not yet free and over-enthusiastic attempts to do this could cause scars or pain. In desert countries the risk of sand under the foreskin may justify circumcision. (*See* BALANITIS.)

Cirrhosis.

Disease of the liver marked by deterioration of the cells and formation of hard scar tissue. There are many causes. (*See* ALCOHOLISM.)

Cleft Palate.

During development of a baby in the womb the roof of

the mouth is split, and the upper lip has two splits which normally join before birth. If the roof of the mouth fails to join the condition is known as cleft palate; the lip as hare-lip. These may interfere with feeding; a prompt operation should rectify. Occasionally further surgery is required and there should be little problem with speech.

Cold. (*Coryza*)

A frequent illness in civilized communities due to virus infection; not dangerous in itself but occasionally the fore-runner of serious bronchitis, pneumonia, etc. (See below.) If you have a cold avoid mixing as viruses spread in crowded, muggy conditions. Low temperature does not seem to cause colds and probably their prevalence is due to living together in *poorly ventilated, over-heated conditions*. The best treatment is a day or two in bed. Two soluble aspirins or Paracetamol may be taken up to four times a day. Keep the patient warm, diet light, fluids plentiful. Lemon or honey drinks soothe, whisky is a pleasant night-cap but little more. Gargles like glycerin and thymol may prevent secondary infection. The virus does not respond to antibiotics so do not request these unless you suffer asthma, bronchitis or heart disease. Complications include sinusitis and bronchitis. (*See* ANTRUM, BRONCHITIS *and* CATARRH.) Vitamin C has been tried as a cold preventive. There is no real evidence it is effective but no harm in it.

There is no scientific proof, but avoiding draughts, changing into dry clothing if soaked and avoiding too many late nights *appear* to reduce the incidence of colds, perhaps because resistance is stronger. A cold lasts two weeks if treated and fourteen days if not!

Colic.

Griping intermittent abdominal pain. Originally referred only to pain in the colon (large bowel) but now used to describe sharp periodic pain in many organs. Adults should see a doctor for investigation. Colic as indicated by screaming attacks is common in infants around three months; it usually responds to Merbentyl syrup, 2.5mls (half a teaspoonful) before feeds.

Colitis.

Inflammation of the colon (the large terminal portion of the bowel) (*see* Fig. 1, *page 31*.) Usually associated with abdominal pain, and diarrhoea, accompanied by mucus (slime) or even blood. Two important types are mucous and ulcerative colitis. The former may be associated with nervous stress while the latter which is more serious and debilitating may have an allergic basis. Many drugs are available to help; a recent advance is the use of disodium cromoglycate. Occasionally part of the bowel may have to be removed if colitis persists and an ileostomy is performed. (*See* ILEOSTOMY.)

Colostomy.

The surgical manufacture of a new opening of the large bowel on the surface of the abdomen. This is necessary after removal of a large part of diseased bowel. The motions are discharged into disposable polythene bags, which has made life much easier. Improved surgical methods have resulted in regular and predictable bowel action in many cases, so the sufferer rarely needs to tolerate a soiled bag for long. Earlier problems of erratic motions and odour have largely been overcome. The Colostomy Welfare Group exists to help sufferers with this condition. (*See* ILEOSTOMY.)

Coma.

A state of unconsciousness, lasting more than a few minutes, from which the patient cannot be roused even by powerful stimulation. There are many causes such as overdose of drugs or alcohol, diseases or injuries to the brain. The layman should send at once for medical aid. The patient should be made comfortable and kept warm. *Give nothing* since trying to force liquids down the throat of an unconscious person will usually result in choking. Anything tight should be removed from the neck, and the patient observed to see if he is breathing. If not, artificial respiration may be necessary. (*See* ASPHYXIA *and* ARTIFICIAL RESPIRATION.)

Concussion.

Brain injury produced by jarring violence to the head which may result in dazing, vomiting or unconsciousness (*see* COMA). Severe concussion may be associated with other injuries such as fractured skull, and is often followed by some loss of memory (*see* AMNESIA) and headaches. Urgently call a doctor and ambulance for a severe head injury. If the patient is unconscious treat until help arrives, as for coma.

Symptoms to take seriously even if the head injury *seems* trivial include being "knocked out" even for a second or so, nausea and vomiting, double vision, pallor and clamminess. In these circumstances the patient should be taken to a hospital casualty department.

Congenital dislocation of the hip.

A few babies are born with dislocated hip joints. Fortunately this is now routinely tested for in the West, and is usually cured after the wearing of a splint for a few months. (*See* LIMP.)

Conjunctivitis.

Inflammation of the delicate membrane lining the eye and the inside of the lids. It results in redness especially at the corners of the eye and watery or sticky discharge. The lids may be stuck together in the mornings. The condition is often due to infection but may also be caused by chemicals or allergy (hay fever). Mild symptoms may respond to bathing with boric acid solution (a pinch to an eyeglass of water) but a *painful* eye needs urgent medical advice as other serious conditions may be present. Any eye problem should always be shown to a doctor. Treatment of the usual infective conjunctivitis is by antibiotic eyedrops.

Conjunctivitis is infectious, so keep children off school for a day or two and their handkerchieves and towels must be kept separate and boiled. (*See also* EYES, EYESIGHT, etc.)

Constipation

This occurs when the bowel motions are hard and passed infrequently or with difficulty. Healthy bowel action is easy and regular although there is a great variation in the frequency of movements – from perhaps twice to thrice daily down to one every three days. What matters is the ease with which the motion is passed.

Lack of roughage and exercise, also the rush to work sometimes ignoring the call to evacuate, are the usual causes of constipation. By the regular use of laxatives the bowels become less sensitive.

Constipation can generally be corrected by a couple of teaspoons of powdered bran sprinkled on a cereal daily, fruit, vegetables, more exercise and time in the morning to accommodate the bowel habit. This can be further helped by two teaspoons of Isogel granules or Dorbanex at night if necessary but do not rely on medicines. Occasional laxatives may be necessary if travelling to where the water or food supply differs. Regular laxatives may be essential for a few but only on medical advice. *Report any persistent change in bowel habits.*

Children after potty training should be encouraged and given time to open the bowels daily after breakfast. Encourage children to eat a diet rich in fruit, fibre and vegetables. *Aperients should not be given to children unless on a doctor's instructions.*

Contraception.
The Pill

Contraception was revolutionised in the 'fifties by the development and use of synthetic progestogens – *see* HORMONES – which act as contraceptives; their main action is to prevent release of the egg to the fallopian tube. They have other complex effects preventing conception, especially when combined with oestrogen – another female hormone.

Family planning is covered by our National Health Service and advice can be obtained from local clinics or many family doctors. Similar arrangements exist abroad.

A medical check is needed before the pill can be prescribed. A history of thrombosis, high blood pressure or recent jaundice rules it out. During diarrhoea or vomiting the pill may pass too quickly to be effective so extra precautions such as the sheath should be used then. Varicose veins or migraine can be made worse. Generally women over 35 should choose another method but *be guided by your doctor.* After starting the pill you need to be seen three-monthly at first for check-up and thereafter once or twice a year.

Most pills are taken once daily for *three* weeks out of four. Take the pill at the same time (usually bedtime) as varying the time can lead to spotting of blood from the vagina. In the *fourth* week there is a small painless "period" when the womb sheds its lining. This prevents "build-up" and provides reassurance that pregnancy has not occurred. Most side effects are minor and explained in leaflets in the packs. *If in doubt about a symptom you must see your doctor.* Extra vitamin B6 can often reverse any lack of sex drive or depression. Check with your doctor if any additional medicines are prescribed. Treatments such as antibiotics or aspirin can reduce effectiveness of the pill. This may be indicated by spotting of blood from the vagina which should not generally happen after the first two months. Take additional precautions (e.g. the sheath) when this happens.

There is a slightly increased risk of blood clotting from the oestrogen component of the pill although risk is less than that in a pregnancy. Risks apply mainly to women over 35 and smokers.

A pill containing progestogen only is suitable for many women, especially those who are breast feeding and the over 35s. The effectiveness is only slightly less; periods may be erratic. This low dose pill may let women continue the pill well into their forties.

"Morning after" – "emergency" only

If unprotected intercourse (e.g. a sheath bursts) occurs, a "morning after" pill can be taken. This usually prevents the fertilised egg from embedding in the womb. Embedding, not fertilisation, is the *hallmark* of pregnancy, so this method may be counted contraceptive and not abortive. This pill must be taken within twelve hours of intercourse and a family planning clinic or doctor *must* be *urgently* consulted. The dose of hormone in the "morning after" pill is high so this method must be reserved for rare "emergency" use. An I.U.D. (see next paragraph) inserted within four or five days of intercourse acts similarly.

Copper or plastic device (I.U.D.)

Many women do not like taking tablets on a long term basis and insertion of a copper or plastic device into the womb may be their ideal solution. Insertion is not painful when done by a *trained* doctor – and some types (including the Copper 7) are suitable for women who have not had a baby. The intra uterine device (I.U.D.) once in place, needs no attention from the patient but needs regular clinic checks (annually unless otherwise instructed).

The I.U.D. is not quite as reliable as the pill and may cause heavier periods. A few women are unable to retain them and tend to expel them with cramping pains shortly after insertion. One expensive type of I.U.D. incorporates a hormone so that the periods are kept light.

With the new advances in hormones it tends to be forgotten that the simple barrier methods are still very effective if used properly.

The Sheath

The sheath (condom) has a success rate comparable to the I.U.D. if combined with a sperm killing chemical. It is more convenient for the woman to take responsibility for the chemical which can be a pessary such as "Orthoform" or a jelly like "Orthogynol". The sheath is also valuable in that it affords some protection against venereal disease whereas the pill has probably contributed to its spreading.

The Cap Method

There is a similar success rate for the female barrier methods of diaphragm or cervical cap also combined with chemicals. These caps must be fitted by a doctor and checked at regular intervals. Some kinds are shown in fig. 4.

Chemical methods alone are not reliable although Delfen Foam is more effective than most.

The Safe Period (Rhythm Method)

The method accepted by Roman Catholics. Unfortunately it has not lived up to early hopes. Being natural it is the perfect birth control but *for its unreliability*. Nevertheless for couples who want, say a 2½ year gap between children but who would not worry were the gap only 12 to

FIG. 4   Contraception cap
W Womb   C Cap   V Vagina

20 months, or for newly married people hoping to wait a few years before parenthood, but whom an earlier conception would not distress, it is excellent. Also, *as an additional method to another*, e.g. the sheath, it has value. The method is based on the fact that the ovum is expected to be released by the ovary about 14 days *before* (note *before*) the first day of the next period. As the ovum can only be fertilised by the sperm for a day or two, in *theory*, all other dates are safe. In practice, intercourse should be avoided for, say, five days before the expected ovulation date, and the expected date, plus three more days, i.e. a total of nine days, (five + one + three). Checks to be sure the woman has periods of regular length (e.g. 28 days) are essential to arrive at what should be the safe dates. Sadly the ovulation is not always regular, and sometimes a second egg is released the next day. At other times ovulation may be early or late for several reasons. Thus the method is not very safe. There are, however, several ways in which greater certainty can be employed but all this is beyond our scope. The Catholic Marriage Advisory Council do a booklet "Natural Family Planning" which gives the latest information. The B.M.A. sell a booklet "Contraception Choice Not Chance".

The Family Planning Association or the equivalent in most lands, are able to help with birth control problems as should your doctor.

The Sponge Method

Widely used years ago but out of fashion. A new dense chemical impregnated sponge is expected to be on the market soon, so keep in touch with your doctor or Family Planning Association in U.K. or similar Associations overseas.

Withdrawal

Coitus interruptus (where the man withdraws from the vagina just before ejaculation) although not completely satisfactory either for sexual harmony or as a method of contraception, is widely practised. It is not a safe method partly because the man often withdraws too late; it is almost impossible not to sometimes, despite what some men imagine. More important – sperms can be present in the urethra before ejaculation.

Sterilisation

Many couples are turning to sterilisation when they think their family is complete. This allows the woman to leave off the pill before the age at which most of the complications occur. It also avoids the problems of heavy periods caused by the I.U.D. in the forties at a stage when the monthly losses tend to be greater. The couple must think the implications through and usually have no regrets. Never forget that circumstances could arise in which you may want to have children again.

Convulsion.

Loss of consciousness with twitching or jerking movement of part or all the body; often known as a "fit". Fits sometimes occur in young children with high temperature, and under these conditions are not necessarily serious. Children who have had one feverish convulsion should be given soluble aspirin and tepid sponging during any subsequent feverish illness such as tonsillitis or a heavy cold. The

FIG. 5 Sterilisation
P Penis   T Testicle   TT Tied
sperm tube (vasectomy)   T Tied off
Fallopian tube   W Womb   O Ovary

danger time is after four p.m. (1600 hours) when temperatures start to rise for the night. If a fit does occur lie the child on his side in a place where he cannot harm himself on furniture, etc. Most feverish fits last only a few minutes but the doctor should be called urgently in case the twitching persists and requires a sedative injection. Feverish fits generally cease by the age of five. (*See* EPILEPSY.)

Corns.

Small areas of painful, compressed thickened skin usually on the toes and largely due to ill-fitting shoes. Corn pads and salt water soaks ease the pain but the best treatment may be skilled chiropody by a Chiropodist (State Registered in the U.K.).

Coronary Thrombosis.

A type of "heart attack" in which a blood vessel (coronary artery) supplying the heart becomes blocked by a clot. (*See* ANGINA.) There is pain in the centre of the chest sometimes radiating to the left arm or jaw. The victim may fall, feel faint and clammy or have difficulty in breathing. Occasionally pain is the only symptom and the patient may not feel ill. The pain is "dull", "heavy", or constricting – never sharp. Any sudden central chest pain especially if accompanied by any of the above symptoms needs urgent medical attention.

If the patient has collapsed urgent transfer to hospital is necessary via the ambulance service. Also call a doctor, in case the ambulance is delayed. If you suspect the heart has stopped in a previously healthy person (confirm by ear directly over the left nipple area) a sharp blow of the fist over the breast bone (centre of the chest) will occasionally re-start it. Artificial respiration should be given if there is no sign of breathing (*see* ASPHYXIA *and* ARTIFICIAL RESPIRATION). Otherwise the patient should be left where he is, if possible, covered by a blanket or coat and left flat if he is conscious, on the left side if unconscious and slightly propped up only if in breathing difficulty. *Do not try to sit him up.* In less severe cases call your doctor urgently. He will decide whether to look after the sufferer at home or admit him to hospital. In hospital the heart beat can be continuously monitored by an electrocardiograph (E.C.G.) so that any complications are spotted immediately and treated. Such complex treatment may not be needed and the main treatment is rest.

The blocked artery stops blood containing oxygen and nourishment reaching part of the heart muscle. This area of muscle is damaged and is eventually replaced by a firm scar.

During recovery the aim is to ensure that the remaining healthy heart muscle can cope.

Patients found to have high blood pressure or cholesterol levels are put on a low animal fat diet and given appropriate tablets. They should stop smoking (*see* SMOKING, *page 15*) and aim to lose any excess weight. Alcohol, a mild heart poison, should be avoided.

Convalescent patients should aim at gradually increasing exercise such as walking, or special exercises provided in a heart clinic gymnasium, until restored to normal activities.

Previously inactive subjects should walk when possible and keep car driving to a minimum. Most can resume sexual intercourse some eight to twelve weeks after an uncomplicated coronary.

There is no sure way to prevent a coronary thrombosis. Plenty of exercise, a low fat and low sugar diet, no smoking, little or no alcohol, a free and easy attitude, all help, but some families have a worse record than others. If you have a bad family record for heart disease it is worth asking your doctor to check your blood pressure and blood cholesterol. If the record is good forget the subject and enjoy life.

Cot Death.

The term for sudden death in babies under a year, usually around three to five months. No single cause has been found although often the child has apparently had a trivial "cold" for a few days. Acute allergy has been suggested, but it does seem that in some cases an apparently insignificant infection has suddenly proved fatal. Much support is needed for parents who suffer needless guilt feelings.

Breast fed babies are less likely to get infections and allergy than are the bottle fed so this seems another good reason to promote breast feeding. Solid foods which can cause allergy are best avoided until the baby is six months old.

Coughing Blood. (*See* HAEMOPTYSIS)

Cramp.

A condition due to a painful muscle spasm, often associated with exposure to cold. It may attack swimmers who have been in the water too long. Treat by "straightening" the cramped part and vigorously rubbing the sore muscle to warm it and restore circulation. In hot climates cramp may be due to lack of salt. Taking more salt with the diet may be essential; salt tablets are available for this purpose. Cramp endangers swimmers but is less likely to occur if bathing is postponed 1½ hours after meals. (It is safer to stay within one's depth.) Leg cramps at night are usually associated with poor circulation and respond well to quinine bisulphate tablets which, because of side effects, should be taken only under doctor's orders.

Cretin.

A rare condition in which babies are born with a defective thyroid gland. Early treatment should prevent mental retardation and other abnormalities.

Croup.

A condition resulting from partial obstruction of the larynx (voice box) occurring chiefly in children and characterised by barking cough, hoarseness and breathing difficulty. Infection causes swelling of the larynx lining so that the small air passage becomes blocked. Relief can be obtained in a steamy atmosphere provided by a kettle in the room. Call a doctor if there is any degree of breathing distress. The child tends to grow out of this as the voice box becomes larger and less easily blocked. Experienced mothers can cope with milder attacks on their own by the use of steam. Breathing distress occurring for the first time in a young child needs urgent medical attention.

Cyst.

A collection of fluid in a part of the body. A common cyst in the skin is due to fluid in a blocked oil-producing gland. This is known as a sebaceous cyst or wen and the best treatment is surgical removal – a tiny operation. If left cysts may become infected and cause trouble.

Cystitis.

Medical term for bladder inflammation, usually accompanied by severe pain and frequency in passing water. The bladder lies low in the abdomen and receives the urine from the kidneys. (*See* Fig. 1, *page 00*.) Sometimes germs enter the bladder and cause infection and inflammation.

Cystitis is more common in women because the germs which often cause it come from the bowel; the openings from the bladder and the bowels are closer in the female. To avoid cystitis women should take particular care in their personal hygiene. Some patients find it helps (and saves fuel) to take showers rather than bath (bowel germs are present in static bath water). After emptying the bowels, toilet paper should be employed in a front to back direction; not the reverse. Symptoms often follow sexual intercourse and sufferers should always empty the bladder immediately after intercourse. Patients with symptoms should take a urine sample (the portion caught in midstream) in a sterile container (boiled bottle will do) to their doctor to test. Tests may confirm the usual bowel germ (E. Coli) and antibiotics usually cure. In the meantime plenty of fluids (five to six pints of water daily) and an alkali such as potassium citrate mixture, one tablespoon in half a tumbler of water three times a day, will soothe.

Recurrent attacks or failure to clear might indicate need for specialist investigation.

Some patients with recurrent symptoms never show evidence of germs. The problem may be one of chemicals or rubber sensitivity due to contraceptives, perfumed bath products or deodorants.

Some women fear venereal disease as symptoms often occur in the early months of intercourse. Although this is usually not the cause they should voice these worries to their doctor or attend a special clinic so that a few extra simple tests can be performed.

After the menopause the tissues around the bladder exit and front passage become delicate and easily inflamed so that cystitis may again become common. Oestrogen creams often help the other treatments here.

Even a single attack of cystitis in a child needs specialist investigation to ensure that infection is not passing upwards into the kidney tubes leading from the bladder.

D

Deafness.

There are two types. One is due to inadequacy of the nerve endings in the ear (cochlea) and the other is due to impaired conduction of sound through the "soundbox" of the ear. Nerve deafness may be present at birth or result from head injury, exposure to excessive noise (in industry, airports, noisy warehouse, music, shooting, the "pop" world, etc.) and virus infections. It is also the deafness which occurs gradually with advancing years although it can affect some individuals earlier in life than average. *Noise-produced deafness should be preventable*. It is regrettable that many workers in noisy occupations fail to wear the protective ear pads provided. Otherwise the only treatment is to amplify residual hearing by a hearing aid. The National Health Service now provides neat behind-the-ear aids.

In the U.K. babies are tested for hearing at seven months and thereafter at pre-school and infant school checks. If you have any doubts about your child's hearing tell your doctor at once so that further tests can be carried out. Normal hearing is necessary for the development of speech.

Conduction deafness can be due to various conditions of the middle and outer ear. Germs may enter the ear, (connected by a tube with the throat), following a cold or other infection. These will cause inflammation and temporary deafness. Nowadays antibiotics will cure the infections but occasionally catarrhal or glue-like fluid and deafness persists. The patient – usually a child – needs to be checked after treatment for middle ear infection in case this fluid needs draining by a specialist. Sometimes special tubes known as grommets are used. There must be no swimming whilst the tubes are in place. Intermittent or doubtful deafness should be taken seriously in a child as the condition is likely to be due to fluid or "glue" which may not settle spontaneously.

Although the eardrum may perforate in an infection it usually heals quickly with modern treatment. Occasionally a perforation may not heal and the ear may discharge at intervals for years. The combination of imperfect drum and discharge in the middle ear causes deafness. Some perforations can now be patched surgically. If the small bones in the ear harden (otosclerosis) there is again a form of conduction deafness. This condition worsens in pregnancy and sometimes on the "pill" and these points should be carefully considered by any sufferer. Surgery may help but not always. In several forms of conduction deafness where surgery can do no more the hearing aid has a large part to play.

In severe deafness lip reading may be the best means for communication. Classes are unfortunately few but details can be had from the Royal National Institute for the Deaf.

Syringing the ear is only of value if wax is present in the outer canal. This is common and fortunately easy to cure. (*See* EARACHE, OTITIS MEDIA, TINNITUS *and* WAX.)

Death.

The layman is sometimes confronted with death. One urgent question is, has death occurred, or is there a possibility of help? Urgently check if breathing (even slight) continues, check for heart beats and note if the body is stiff or cold. To test breathing look carefully at the chest to see if it moves; if in doubt, hold a mirror, failing which a piece of glass, close to the mouth and nostrils to see if it becomes clouded. If beating, the heart may be heard by placing one ear on the chest in the region of the left nipple, or the pulse may be felt for on the front of the wrist just below the base of the thumb. If there is no breathing, no heart beat, and particularly if the body is stiff or cold, death has occurred. If there is a sign of life treat the patient as for shock (*see* SHOCK) until medical aid arrives. If necessary the kiss of life must be tried while awaiting help. (*See* ARTIFICIAL RESPIRATION *and* COT DEATH.)

Delirium.

A state of restlessness, the patient being only partly conscious. Delirium usually accompanies a high fever, and the patient may throw himself about, pick at the bedclothes and mutter without ceasing. It may help, if the patient is conscious to give soluble aspirin, and sponge him down with tepid water until the doctor arrives. This will reduce the temperature of the body, and often quieten the patient for a while. A special form of delirium known as *delirium tremens* is associated with alcoholism. (*See* ALCOHOLISM.)

Dementia. (*Senile Dementia*)
Progressive condition of loss of intelligence often found in old age. Poor memory and self-neglect are early signs. Hospital care may eventually be needed. (*See* MENTAL ILLNESS *and* OLD AGE.)

Dentures.
Those who suffer from badly fitting artificial teeth should not put up with them. Return to your dentist and get a good set. If he cannot fit you then change your dentist or get a set made privately.

If you have a good set there should be no need to remove them at night, which is a morale-booster. Wash them night and morning and brush the gums. Some doctors would disagree but millions are not any the worse for retaining them. Small or part plates should be removed while asleep, due to danger of swallowing.

Painful biting may improve as the gums harden. For some foods you may need to use suction (consciously) and your tongue to prevent the teeth tipping forward. Progress to harder foods and ultimately you can aim to eat apples without quartering them.

Depression.
A condition which may include depressed mood, apathy, feelings of guilt, lack of physical energy and disturbed sleep. It always needs urgent attention especially in the early weeks after childbirth. (*See* MENTAL ILLNESS.)

Dermatitis.
Means inflammation of the skin and thus covers practically the whole range of skin diseases. The lay idea that it is a "dirty" condition is false. Common examples are contact

dermatitis due to sensitivity to detergents or metals such as nickel. Barrier creams such as Atrixo and gloves help as does hydrocortisone cream (available only on prescription).

Dextrose.

A form of the quick-acting sugar glucose, available in tablets as Dextrosol and useful to restore energy and prevent sleepiness in long distance drivers. (They are carried by diabetics to ward off sudden falls in blood sugar and prevent coma.)

Dhobie Itch. (*See* ATHLETE'S FOOT *and* TINEA)

Diabetes.

In diabetes the body is unable to make proper use of carbohydrates or sugary foods. Normally carbohydrates undergo changes in the body with release of energy which the body can use. These changes are controlled by insulin, made by one of the internal glands, the pancreas. (*See* FIG. 1, *page* 31.) In diabetes the pancreas fails to make sufficient insulin so that sugar, instead of being properly used, accumulates. The kidneys try to get rid of this excess sugar so the patient passes more urine than normal, and often has a persistent thirst in consequence. Other symptoms include general ill health, a loss of weight and energy, itching of the skin and a liability to infections such as boils. There are two types of diabetes – one occurring in the young and the other in older obese patients.

The young diabetic always needs regular replacement insulin whereas the older patient may respond to diet restriction only or to diet plus tablets such as chlorpropamide. These allow the patient to make the most of his limited supplies of natural insulin. Insulin must be given by injection since it is destroyed by digestive juices. Most diabetics, (including many doctors!) can lead normal lives with one or two injections daily. They must have regular mealtimes and become familiar with their exercise tolerance, otherwise they tend to plunge into low blood sugar states. Once they and their doctors have got their diet, insulin requirement and exercise balanced, they can live full lives. Feelings of faintness, irritability or lack of concentration can indicate low blood sugar and they always carry glucose tablets for this reason.

Diabetics usually carry a card or wear a medical bracelet stating their condition. If a person is found in a semi-conscious or "drunk" state it is worth checking this. If he is sufficiently conscious to swallow sugar this may bring him round, otherwise urgent medical attention is needed.

Diarrhoea.

A condition in which the stools are abnormally fluid, but is commonly used when the bowels are opened more often than the normal. These conditions often occur together. There are many causes of diarrhoea. In children it may follow over-eating of fruit, but is usually due to infection. For mild diarrhoea it is best to live on liquids only for twenty-four hours e.g. dilute fruit juices or glucose solution – one desertspoon to a pint of water plus a pinch of salt. Mist. kaolin or in the case of children, children's mist. kaolin may control diarrhoea. Follow this by a light diet for the next day or two – no meat, vegetables or whole fruit for three days. If diarrhoea persists, if accompanied by a pain or a raised temperature, see a doctor. Babies (under one year) should be seen early by a doctor as they are suscept-ible to fluid loss and can become dangerously low in body fluid.

Diplopia. (See DOUBLE VISION)

Diphtheria.

A disease, once of world-wide distribution, now largely disappeared from Europe and North America due to vac-cination.

It starts as a throat infection and produces a membrane which may obstruct breathing. It also produces a poison which can damage the heart and nerves.

Any throat infection accompanied by high fever needs medical attention. It is unlikely to be diphtheria in the West but might be tonsillitis requiring penicillin. If there is any reason for suspicion a special test can be made.

Discharge.

Outpouring of fluid from a body opening e.g. from the nose during a cold. One cause of worry is discharge from the sex organs which may be due to veneral infection (*see* GONORRHOEA). There are other causes, especially in women, but any discharge of this nature should receive urgent medical attention. There may be a harmless explanation, but neglect could be serious.

Dislocation.

Occurs when a bone slips out of place. It normally results from violence and may occur at almost any joint. Perhaps the most common is dislocation of the shoulder, when the rounded head of the humerus (the bone in the upper arm) slips out of its hollow in the shoulder. There is acute pain, and the joint becomes fixed. The unskilled should do nothing except make the patient comfortable and get medical help. Attempts to move the dislocated bone may damage the joint and must be avoided. The part affected may be supported, e.g. by a sling or cushion, until the doctor arrives.

Disseminated Sclerosis. (*See* MULTIPLE SCLEROSIS)

Diverticulitis.

Inflammation of the intestine due to small pockets which become irritated and infected forming in the walls of the bowel. Before inflammation and infection occur the condition may be controlled by a diet rich in bran and roughage. Isogel granules and tablets to control bowel spasm can be prescribed.

If infection occurs it can often be cured by antibiotics. Operation is rarely necessary.

Dog Bite (*including rabies*).

To be bitten by a dog can be dangerous because of transfer of infection. The most serious is the disease known as rabies (hydrophobia) which causes madness in dogs. Those bitten often acquire the infection and die painfully. Fortunately, due to quarantine rules, dogs entering the U.K. are isolated under observation for six months to ensure they are not infected. As at 1979 this means there is no rabies in Britain. Sadly the disease has reached Northern Europe and there is a risk it may reach the U.K. This could be due to a misguided animal lover smuggling a pet through the Customs. The animal often bites before the disease is apparent so it is not always easy to make a quick diagnosis.

If abroad where rabies is endemic avoid contact with animals, e.g. dogs, cats and hedgehogs. If scratched or bitten wash the wound with detergent and apply alcohol. Check if the animal has been inoculated against rabies. Tell the owner to let you know if it becomes ill. If no information is available or the animal is a stray go immediately to the nearest doctor as a course of vaccination may have to be started. *Do not wait for symptoms as the disease is always fatal once symptoms develop*.

Apart from such serious considerations any dog bite may go septic due to commonly occurring germs. All bites should be treated promptly with an antiseptic. (*See* ABRASION). For severe bites, consult a doctor. Tetanus is another potentially fatal disease which can be acquired from a cut or dog bite. Everyone can be immunised against tetanus so that this problem need not arise. Check with your doctor that your immunity is up-to-date.

If attacked by a dog it usually pays to face it and talk to it. You may have to shout at it, but that is better than trying to outdistance it by running away. If you have a stick or a chair point in at the dog's eyes. Small dogs can be biters and in self-defence you may have to kick them away.

Dotage. (*See* OLD AGE)

Double Vision. (*Diplopia*)
Diplopia may be due to weakness or lack of balance of the eye muscles (*see* SQUINT). Occasionally it may be due to illness so anyone who sees double should consult a doctor urgently. Glasses may be all that are required, but if there is a serious cause the sooner it is dealt with the better.

Drinking. (*See* ALCOHOLISM, ADDICTION, *and page* 16.)

Dropsy. (*See* OEDEMA)

Drowning.

Drowning occurs when enough oxygen cannot reach the lungs following submersion in water. Without a continual supply from the air the tissues of the body rapidly die. In drowning, therefore, it is vital to restore normal breathing if there is the slightest chance of recovery. **SEE ARTIFICIAL RESPIRATION, page 35.**

Drug.

Any substance which affects the working of the body, and is used in treatment. The term is *not* restricted to substances which cause drowsiness or addiction.

Drug Addiction and abuse.

In all types of drug addiction the body becomes dependent on more and more quantities of drug with ever more damage from side effects. Young people should realise that there is nothing clever in getting involved in pot parties where even stronger drugs may be passed around. Although at the present time it is not certain whether long term effects of pot are as medically damaging as those of alcohol or nicotine, it is almost certain that some untoward effects will be demonstrated with continued use and the risk is not worth taking. A danger in joining in group activities is of being introduced, perhaps accidentally, to a very disturbing drug such as L.S.D. This produces hallucinations (the trip) which can be nightmarish or euphoric. Unfortunately, during a euphoric sense of power people have jumped from buildings under the impression that they could fly. The "low" trips can produce a nightmarish variety of depression which can persist for months after the original dose. A patient of mine had this experience after some L.S.D. was "planted" in his beer. He needed about a year of psychiatric treatment to regain his equanimity.

Another killer is heroin, often used with cocaine. Here the increasing physical dependence and complications commonly lead to death if treatment is not started early. Tragic mistakes occur as when a man foolishly injects his girl friend with a dose that he is taking, forgetting that *he* has *worked his way up to what is a lethal dose for a newcomer.*

Some people seem to be more prone to addiction than others and can rapidly become hooked. No-one should get involved with even the mildest of pot smoking or pill swapping groups. You may be the unlucky one. Only foolish people run such risks, which can harm for life, or kill.

Duodenal Ulcer.

The duodenum is part of the small intestine leading out of the stomach. An ulcer is a gap in the lining of the duodenum so that the sensitive underlayers are exposed. Due to imbalance in the digestive juices reaching the duodenum from the stomach the lining becomes inflamed and later eroded to form an ulcer. Smoking, irregular, infrequent meals and mental stress predispose to ulcers.

A substance called histamine is important in controlling the acidity of stomach juice and its release is controlled by certain nerves. Nicotine and adrenalin (the "stress hormone") affect histamine release. A useful new drug to treat ulcers (cimetidine) acts by blocking histamine release. Other drugs which can heal ulcers are based on liquorice extracts.

The progress of ulcers can be checked by barium X-rays and a flexible telescope for direct viewing into the stomach.

Typical symptoms are pain which remains fairly localized a little above the navel. It comes on an hour or so after meals; it may last for the best part of an hour, sometimes with a feeling of sickness and occasionally vomiting. Flatulence (wind) is common. Ulcers require medical treatment, for if they continue there is a danger of internal bleeding or of the ulcer spreading through the wall and causing a perforation. Bed rest is still useful in severe cases. A light diet is usual for a week or two but thereafter there is no need for restrictions other than the avoidance of fried and spicy foods. A patient will find items to be avoided by trial and error. The important point is regular, frequent meals. Alkali tablets such as "Roter" may help, as do tablets to relieve stomach spasms such as Probanthine and Merbentyl. The mainstay of treatment however is the newer type "healing tablet" combined with *giving up smoking* and avoiding stress.

If the ulcer will not heal, and pain is severe, an operation may be needed. Normally this presents no difficulties in skilled hands.

Dysentery.

Infectious disease of the intestines caused by bacteria which give rise to inflammation. The germs are spread by contaminated food and water supplies, etc. The disease is rare in the U.K. but common in hot climates. Symptoms are diarrhoea, which may be accompanied by a little blood, colicky pain in the stomach and usually fever. Attention to fluid requirements, bowel slowing tablets, and appropriate antibiotics will usually cut short an attack. See your doctor.

Another type of dysentery found in the East is caused by a parasite which burrows in the wall of the intestine. This is known as *amoebic dysentery*, and although the symptoms are usually less severe it runs a more chronic course than bacterial dysentery and is often difficult to cure. Travellers from the East with persistent bowel symptoms need specialised investigation.

Dyslexia.

"Word blindness" – in which a person of normal intelligence has difficulty in learning to read. In U.K. patients can be referred to a few special centres.

Dysmenorrhoea.

Painful periods can be due to many causes. In girls the neck of the womb is unstretched and the slight contractions during menstruation pull on the cervix causing pain. This improves after the first day and usually disappears if the patient has a child. Girls who have unusually severe pain may be producing high levels of substances known as Prostaglandins. Painkillers such as soluble aspirin, Indocid and "Ponstan" which neutralise the effects of Prostaglandins may help. More helpful still is one of a variety of hormones known as progestogens. Painful periods in middle age or at other times may be due to other gynaecological disorders. If they persist consult your doctor.

Dyspareunia.

The term given to painful sexual intercourse. In the woman there is usually some difficulty the first time intercourse takes place. The entrance to the vagina (female passage) is more or less sealed by a membrane known as the hymen, and this must be broken before full penetration can take place. Sometimes where early attempts have been clumsy or painful the woman becomes frightened or apprehensive so that subsequent union is difficult for her and her partner. Girls who dreamed intercourse would be fabulous (it can be but not at first) often find the required adjustments a bit of a shock. If the man is patient, encouraging and loving, above all loving, and gives his girl time, perhaps even days, before entering *fully*, normally all should come right within weeks.

In some cases dyspareunia is due to disease or inflammation of the vagina or pelvic organs. Where dyspareunia comes on suddenly after previously painless intercourse medical investigation is needed. A few marriages are doomed because the couples are for one reason or another unable to establish a proper physical union, and it is vital that advice should be sought if there is continued difficulty. (*See* FRIGIDITY.)

Dyspepsia.

A rather loose term covering different types of indigestion. Dyspepsia usually implies discomfort and flatulence following meals. It may be due to over-indulgence (*see* ACIDOSIS) or at other times associated with internal disorders, such as ulcers (*see* DUODENAL ULCER) or gallstones.

E

Earache.

May be due to several causes. Infection of the middle ear (*see* OTITIS MEDIA) may follow a cold. Small boils known as furuncles sometimes develop in the canal leading from the outer ear to the ear drum and are very painful. They require medical advice. The amount of wax produced varies from person to person but is sometimes sufficient to block the ear completely and causes discomfort. When this happens it may be removed by a doctor or nurse using a syringe. The wax should be softened with almond oil or Waxsol for a few days first. Earache is often a great worry in children and if it does not quickly settle down or is associated with any fever, the child should always be seen by a doctor. Antibiotics may be needed and careful follow-up by the doctor is necessary to prevent complications like deafness and mastoiditis. For temporary relief disprin and warmed ear drops of "Audax" or "Auralgicin" are helpful.

FIG. 6   The ear
A   Auricle   B   Canal leading to ear
drum   C   Ossicles   D   Cavity of
middle ear   E   Ear drum   F   Mastoid
process containing air cells
G   Cochlea   H   Auditory nerve
I   Eustachian tube

Temporary earache can afflict airline passengers. When the aircraft ascends, passengers may notice their ears "popping", but this does not result in pain.

When an aircraft descends, the pressure in the cabin increases and the eardrums are pushed inwards, which can produce pain. The remedy is to "clear the ears", which is achieved by yawning, swallowing, chewing, sucking, wiggling the jaw, or by closing the mouth and blowing against a nose which is pinched firmly shut. Babies can be helped by being given a drink.

It is unwise to fly with nasal congestion (e.g. cold or hay fever, etc.), and those who suffer should consult a doctor, as should anyone whose discomfort persists more than a few hours after landing. (*See* DEAFNESS, MASTOID *and* OTOR-RHOEA.)

Ectopic Pregnancy.

A pregnancy which occurs outside the womb. The womb is connected by means of two tubes with the ovaries. The female egg or ovum passes down these tubes (the fallopian tubes) into the womb and when fertilization takes place the ovum normally lodges in the uterus. It occasionally happens that the fertilized ovum lodges in one of the tubes. When this occurs there is no room for the ovum to grow, so that trouble soon develops. Often there is pain in the lower part of the abdomen on one side and brown discharge or slight bleeding from the vagina. If the condition continues the fallopian tube may burst. The symptoms often occur soon after a missed period before pregnancy is confirmed so in the event of pain and brown discharge contact your doctor without delay even if you are not sure you are pregnant. The treatment of an ectopic pregnancy is by operation to remove the bursting tube. Both ovaries and one healthy tube are left so fertility is not greatly affected.

Eczema.

A chronic skin disease in which the most prominent features are redness, soreness, weeping and irritation. It is often seen over the knuckles, wrists and elbows, and may be associated with widespread dryness and scaling of the skin. The condition is due to sensitivity of the skin (*see* ALLERGY) and similar conditions such as asthma or hay fever may be met with in the same family.

Eczema is common in babies, and sometimes food such

as eggs or chocolate may be found responsible. The "foreign" protein in cow's milk can cause allergy in babies and may even be responsible for long term problems. Breast feeding largely avoids this problem and if there is a family history of allergy, cow's milk should not be given during the first year of life if possible. Fortunately many babies will grow out of the tendency to develop eczema. The treatment of *established* eczema is difficult, and often calls for patience in the doctor and patient. If a cause such as food allergy can be found its elimination will go far towards curing, but often it is difficult to discover, or there may be many causes. Eczema patients should never use soap. Oily preparations such as oilatum can be used for washing. Ointments incorporating coal tar, hydrocortisone or urea are helpful whilst dry skin patches may respond to lubricating creams such as E45 or Unguentum (Merck). Treatment has to be continued as long as the eczema persists.

Electric Shock.

The danger from the passage of electricity through the body is threefold. Firstly, there may be a burn at the points where the electric current enters and leaves. This may be treated on general lines. (*See* BURNS). Secondly, the current has a paralysing effect on the nervous system and the heart. The victim may be stunned into unconsciousness and the heart may stop beating and breathing cease. Thirdly, strong muscular spasms are provoked which are damaging and may lead to temporary paralysis and stiffness.

When a person suffers electric shock first make certain that contact with the current is broken. Do not touch the victim with your hand or you will suffer a shock yourself, but use some non-conducting material, a stick, a wooden chair, a cushion – something dry and *not* containing metal. Next see if the victim is breathing. If he is he may be kept warm and made comfortable but if not apply artificial respiration until medical help arrives. If you suspect that the heart has stopped (confirm by ear directly over the left nipple area), a sharp blow of the fist directly over the breast bone (centre of the chest) will occasionally re-start it. (*See* ARTIFICIAL RESPIRATION *page* 35.)

Electric shocks are best prevented, and great care with

switches, etc., especially in *bathrooms* (for water acts as a conductor) is recommended. "Pull" switches should always be used for electric lights in bathrooms. Electric fires should never be used there, except for the high wall-fitted types with pull switches.

Great care should be taken in the kitchen so that damp hands are never used to deal with switches and plugs. "Safety" wall sockets should always be used especially where there are children in the house. All electrical gadgets should be checked by an expert at the slightest sign of defects and house wiring should meet modern safety standards; improvements should be undertaken by qualified electricians only.

Electrocardiogram. *(E.C.G.)* Electrical tracing of heart activity which alters in heart disease and is useful in detecting certain types of illness e.g. coronary thrombosis.

Electro Convulsive Therapy. *(E.C.T.)*
The passage of a tiny electric current through the brain in carefully measured doses to help serious depressive illness and some forms of schizophrenia. This would normally induce convulsions but the patients are given muscle relaxants to prevent this. Although there is much controversy about its use on the grounds that permanent physical damage may be done, it seems to be life-saving in severe depression where other treatments have failed; in these cases there is a high risk of suicide as the patient's feelings of misery are so great that life does not seem worth living. There is usually some memory loss immediately after treatment but this improves with time. I have known many who have had this treatment years ago and they now seem perfectly well. (*See* MENTAL ILLNESS.)

Electroencephalogram. *(E.E.G.)*
Electrical tracing of the "brain waves" helpful in confirming the diagnosis of epilepsy and other diseases.

Embolism.
A clot of blood or other particle carried round the blood stream may lodge in a blood vessel and block it. This cuts

off the blood supply to the organ in question causing tissue damage. Thus a cerebral embolism is a blood clot lodged in one of the arteries of the brain and is one cause of a stroke. (*See* STROKE.) Sometimes the clot can be dispersed by urgent treatment and frequently anti-coagulant tablets are prescribed to prevent further emboli.

Emphysema.

Swelling and bursting of the delicate terminal air passages in the lungs. It is often associated with narrowing of the large air tubes (bronchi) as in chronic bronchitis. The passage of oxygen into the blood is less effective than it should be and shortness of breath results.

Empyema.

An empyema can be described as an abscess on the lung (*see* ABSCESS). The lung is enclosed in a double layer of membrane which protects it, and if the lung becomes inflamed fluid may form between the layers. If germs spread from the lung this fluid may become infected and an empyema has developed. This may happen following pneumonia but nowadays antibiotics generally clear a chest infection before this stage. If pus does collect it may be drained by a tube inserted into the chest.

Encephalitis.

The medical term for inflammation of the brain; a serious condition due to infection by germs – usually the small germs known as viruses. It may occur alone or as a complication of a general illness such as measles; this is one good reason for immunisation against the disease in the second year of life (the risk of encephalitis from the vaccine is much smaller than that from the disease itself). The patient with encephalitis is seriously ill, and may be unconscious or delirious. Treatment is by steriods in the form of ACTH and the outlook for permanent recovery is fairly good.

Endometriosis.

One cause of painful periods. In this condition the menstrual flow tends to run backwards so that fragments of the shed womb lining reach the Fallopian tubes and the ovaries, rather than being completely voided into the vagina. One type of ovarian cyst may form (chocolate cyst) and resultant abdominal pain and possible infertility, require medical attention. Treatment is by hormones and by removal of the cysts. (*See* DYSMENORRHOEA *and* OVARIAN CYST.)

Enuresis. *(Bed wetting)*

A troublesome and common complaint in children. The age a child gains control of the bladder varies considerably; but by the age of four night control is generally achieved. The child only gains voluntary control of his bladder around eighteen months and the ability to use the toilet alone around two to two and a half years. Although regular "potting" of a baby before this age may save wet nappies this is not "training" as no true bladder control is involved. The main help that a mother can give the eighteen month child is to offer the pot after meals, on coming indoors, after walking, etc., but to abandon the attempt after two minutes if there is no response. She should be ready to produce the pot and help the child onto it if he indicates his need but she must also be philosophically prepared for a lot of refusals, false alarms and general messing about. When day-time control is achieved "potting" the child last thing at night may induce night-time dryness. By two and a half the child may co-operate in using a bedside potty, when the night nappy may be discarded. It should not be left off too soon as "accidents" discourage the child and make matters worse. The child will always gain bladder control day and night in his own good time provided that he is given a chance to do so and that he has no undue emotional upsets.

If a child of four is constantly wetting the bed ask your doctor to check his water in case infection is the cause. Usually there is no abnormality and the child gains control a little later. Persistent "dribbling" as opposed to a series of small floods always requires urgent medical investigation.

Some families seem to have "immature" bladders in that many members gain night control very late in childhood. Most doctors will offer treatment at four and a half to five years. Undue restriction of fluids is not helpful and can be cruel. Children may temporarily start wetting the bed again (after being dry) during a family upheaval or hospital admission. Reassurance (and not scolding) is required. The few teenagers who still, to their dismay, wet the bed regularly can be consoled that the condition will definitely clear eventually, as it is virtually unknown in married adults. (*See* INCONTINENCE.)

Epilepsy.

A disease in which the patient suffers from recurrent fits. It appears to be due to inherent electrical instability in the brain, so that every so often there is a sudden release of energy. The instability may be caused by head injury or disease. Often there is no obvious reason and this type of epilepsy begins early in life and tends to run in families. There are many types of epilepsy. In childhood the commonest is *petit mal* in which lapses of consciousness lasting only a few seconds occur. These may be very frequent and scarcely noticeable to the onlooker. They are important as a reason for poor progress or apparent inattentiveness at school. E.E.G. *(see page 90)* helps confirm the diagnosis.

Children may also have *grand mal* which is the commonest form in adults. Often the patient has warning before this type of fit occurs. He sees flashes of light, or may experience some peculiar sensations, known as the aura. Following this there is often a cry and the patient falls unconscious. The body is stiff and rigid, but after a short while rapid jerking movements occur which gradually diminish. The patient goes blue in the face, and may bite his tongue or pass water. During the fit it is best to do as little as possible. If the patient can be caught as he falls injury may be prevented. He should be allowed to lie flat until the fit is over, the neck should be examined to see that it is not constricted by tight clothing, and if anything suitable is available, such as a rolled-up handkerchief, it may be pushed between the teeth to prevent injury to the tongue. After the fit the patient should be put to bed, and he will often sleep. This type of seizure is similar to the feverish convulsion in childhood. (*See* CONVULSION.)

A doctor must be called at the onset of any convulsion in children so that he can, if necessary, give an injection to stop it; prolonged fits can be dangerous. Most adults come out of a fit spontaneously but medical aid must be sought if it persists more than ten minutes. Anticonvulsive medicines can bring about a great reduction in frequency of fits, or even eliminate them. An epileptic may hold a driving licence if he has not had a daytime fit for two years. A heavy goods vehicle licence can never be granted to anyone with a history of even one fit (other than infantile feverish convulsions).

In general, epileptics should lead as full a life as possible, but they must avoid occupations in which a fit would prove dangerous such as driving, window cleaning, or proximity to moving machinery. Ill-informed prejudice against epileptics by employers is to be deprecated. Many doctors have controlled epilepsy themselves. Guidance may be had from the British Epilepsy Association (ask your doctor for the address).

Episiotomy.

Small cut sometimes made under local anaesthetic at the outlet of the vagina, to aid delivery of the baby's head during birth. It avoids overstretching of the muscles and prevents a larger tear; it is stitched up painlessly also under local anaesthetic.

Erysipelas.

A spreading skin infection similar to cellulitis (*see* CELLULITIS). In erysipelas, however, the streptococcal infection spreads within the skin instead of just beneath. The treatment is penicillin.

Erythema.

Redness of the skin, a feature of many rashes and children's illnesses.

Euthanasia.

Means easy or happy death. There are well-meaning people who feel that the individual should be granted the right when incurably ill to ask for release from life at the stage he deems appropriate. The means envisaged is usually a painless injection of a lethal dose of opiate or similar. Euthanasia is illegal.

Strangely, the idea is more popular with younger healthy people who witness what they see as the disintegration and degradation of a person they once loved. The patient himself although perhaps a believer in euthanasia rarely seems to feel that the "right" moment has come. Hospices such as St. Christopher's have brought hope of a pain-free and a fulfilling life to the incurably ill. These patients live every day to the full and accept death on its own terms.

Eyes (Eyesight).

Care of the eyes is important. Inflammation may be due to many causes. Eyes becoming red and irritable, particularly towards the end of the day, are probably being strained. Possibly there may be a slight irregularity in the lens which makes the focussing of light on the back of the eye difficult. The lens may be too flat, which makes the focussing of distant objects easy, but near vision difficult – the condition of long sightedness or *hypermetropia.* If the lens is too curved there is *myopia* or short sightedness; while if the lens is irregular, being too curved in one direction and too flat in another, the condition is described as *astigmatism.* All require glasses or contact lenses.

Various germs can set up inflammation and discharge in the lining of the eye – known as *conjunctivitis* (*see* CONJUNCTIVITIS). If the inflammation does not subside quickly a doctor should be consulted.

Strong sunlight can also cause inflammation, and the eyes should be protected by dark (polarised lens) glasses during the summer, especially at the seaside where the glare can be strong. Misuse of an ultraviolet (sunlight) lamp can cause severe inflammation. Always use the goggles provided and follow the time exposure instructions minutely.

Another cause of irritation is a small particle lodging in the eye. The eye containing a "foreign body" should on no account be rubbed, as this may damage the delicate membrane. The lids should be held open and the eye carefully inspected – under the top lid with the patient looking down, and under the lower lid while looking up. If the particle can be seen it should be gently removed with a wisp of cotton wool or the corner of a clean soft handkerchief. Sometimes

1. Normal Vision
The light from an outside object is brought to a focus accurately on the sensitive retina at the back of the eyeball.

2. Hypermetropia (Long sightedness)
The eyeball is too short or the lens is too weak, so that the light comes to a focus *behind* the retina. Distant objects can be seen more clearly than near ones. Convex glasses are required to correct this error.

3. Myopia (Short sightedness)
the eyeball is too long or the lens is too powerful, so that the light comes to a focus *in front of* the retina. Near objects can be seen more clearly than distant ones. Concave glasses are required to correct this error.

4. Astigmatism
Either the eyeball or the lens is irregular so that light is brought to a focus at different levels in different parts of the eye. Special glasses have to be made to correct the individual error in astigmatism.

FIG. 7   Defective vision
A   Retina   B   Lens   C   Pupil

gently pulling the upper lid over the lower will remove the particle. Often holding the head over a basin of clean water, opening and closing the eye lids under the water can get rid of a particle in the eye. If the particle cannot be seen or moved the patient should be taken to the doctor.

At times the ducts may be blocked causing watery eyes. These can sometimes be cleared by a doctor in a minute or two.

Two important causes of *painful* red eyes are *glaucoma* (*see* GLAUCOMA) and inflammation of the iris (*see* IRITIS). Among warning signs in glaucoma are episodes of mistiness of vision and haloes round lights. These or *any type of sudden visual disturbance indicate the need for urgent investigation.*

Most people probably need glasses around 50. It is unwise to delay being tested if any difficulties are experienced; thereafter have eyesight professionally checked as required, probably every five years.

A doctor should be seen for any pain, sticky discharge, disturbance of vision or persistently red or watery eyes. (*See* ARTERITIS, CATARACT *and* PINK EYE.)

F

Fainting.

A momentary loss of consciousness for which there are many causes. Most faints are not serious and quickly pass. Their cause is often emotional. Some people faint at the sight of blood, others in church or on receiving bad news. These factors cause a temporary upset in the nervous control of the circulation which results in the faint. People vary in their make-up, and some go through life without fainting, while others faint readily. It can be much reduced by the advice to wiggle the toes continuously – thus aiding blood return from the legs to the heart. The person who faints should be kept flat. Nothing more is required, and *it is unwise to try to force fluids (brandy, etc.) down the throat, as this may cause choking.* For a *feeling* of faintness sit and put the head between the knees as far down as possible until the feeling passes.

In a few cases fainting may be a symptom of illnesses such as ANAEMIA or occasionally heart disease. In general a single faint, particularly where there is some emotional cause or in heat, should not be cause for alarm. If, however, a patient faints repeatedly and apparently without reason a doctor must be consulted to see if there is any underlying cause.

Festering. (*See* ABSCESS)

Fever.
The temperature of the human body is carefully regulated, and under normal circumstances varies little. It is normally about 98° Fahrenheit or 37° Centigrade and should not exceed 98.4°F. When the body is attacked by germs a complicated defence system comes into play, and one of the body's reactions is to increase temperature. This serves two purposes. Firstly, the raised temperature is often unsuitable for germs so that they can be more easily destroyed, and, secondly, as the temperature is raised the internal workings of the body are speeded up so that it can work more quickly and efficiently. However, the temperature is only one of many factors to be taken into account and the patient's appearance and other symptoms must be considered. Children "run a temperature" more easily than adults and a mother may be surprised to find that a child with a head cold, not looking particularly ill, has a temperature of 100°F or so. This can be readily treated at home with Disprin unless complications such as earache or chest symptoms occur.

On the other hand a temperature of only 99° to 100°F may be very significant in a patient who feels very unwell especially if there is abdominal pain or vomiting.

As a general rule you need medical advice for a child who has a temperature of 102°F (39°C) and for an adult with a temperature of over 100°F (38°C) but again it is the severity of the symptoms which matters. If your child looks ill, and flushed, is not eating, is complaining of pain or is vomiting you need medical advice regardless of the reading on the thermometer. (*See* HYPOTHERMIA *and* TEMPERATURE).

Fibroids.

Small lumps which develop in the wall of the uterus (womb). They become increasingly common in middle age. Usually the chief symptom is increased loss – "flooding" at the "period". If symptomless they can be left alone but if flooding is severe hysterectomy may be the best treatment (*see* HYSTERECTOMY). Surprisingly, removal of fibroids from the uterus is a more difficult operation than hysterectomy and is only done in women who wish to have further children especially if the fibroids may be causing infertility. Fibroids are not dangerous in themselves, and are not malignant.

Fibrositis. (*See* MUSCULAR RHEUMATISM)

Finger, Septic.

Infection by germs in the soft tissues of the finger is common and can lead to disability if not treated. It may follow a prick or injury, but often the breach in the skin is so small as to escape notice. The finger becomes red, swollen, hot and throbs. Treatment with antibiotics should be started as early as possible. It is always best to consult a doctor for any infection of the finger. If the infection spreads to the base of the nail it will often become chronic and may fail to clear up until the nail is removed. A further danger is that the infection may spread to the tendons which move the finger joints. If this happens the finger may remain permanently stiff.

Fissure-in-Ano.

The opening from the "back passage" is guarded by a circular muscle – the anus. A small split can develop in the overlying skin as a split may develop at the corner of the mouth. This is known as a fissure-in-ano. There is sharp pain each time the bowels are opened, and there may be bleeding. Infection by germs and the fact that the anus is stretched when the bowels are opened make healing difficult. It may respond to keeping the motions soft by a laxative such as "Dorbanex" and to an anaesthetic cream prescribed by your doctor. A small operation may be needed to restore to normal. This condition can often be prevented by avoiding constipation. (*See* CONSTIPATION.)

Fistula.

An abnormal opening between internal organs or between an organ and the surface of the body. A common type is the fistula-in-ano due to infection deep in a fissure-in-ano (see previous article). Treatment is by a minor operation. Pus collects to form an abscess (*see* ABSCESS) and this bursts on to the skin surface close by but *not through* the original fissure. This "abscess" thus has two openings and constitutes a fistula.

Fits. (*See* CONVULSIONS *and* EPILEPSY)

Flat Foot.

The foot has to support the weight of the body for long periods and put up with tremendous stresses during walking, etc. It is constructed on the principle of the arch. There are really two arches formed by the bones of the foot; the longitudinal arch running from front to back, and the transverse arch from side to side. The bones are kept in place by the muscles, tendons and ligaments which bind them together. In "flat foot", the arch sags so that the inner side of the foot touches the ground. It is so common in children that specialists now consider this to be one variety of normal. The foot is painless, arches normally on tiptoe and does not need special exercise or footwear. Where flat foot is painful and caused by arthritis or other diseases orthopaedic help is needed.

Flatulence.

The escape of wind from the digestive tract. The term is usually applied to eructations from the stomach ("belching") but is also used to describe wind from the bowels. Excessive flatulence may be a symptom of disordered digestion (*see* DYSPEPSIA) and is sometimes associated with gall bladder disease or peptic ulcer.

Flooding. (*See* MENORRHAGIA)

Flushing. (*See* MENOPAUSE)

Food Poisoning.

There are two sorts. In the first the food may be poisonous, for example, when poisonous fungus is eaten by mistake. In the second the food is innocent, but is invaded by germs and goes bad; and it is the poison produced by the germs which is responsible for the symptoms. Tinned foods opened and left standing are particularly liable to "go off". The body usually makes every endeavour to get rid of the poison, and severe abdominal pain is followed by vomiting. At a later stage there is usually diarrhoea. Unidentified foods should never be eaten, and one should be suspicious of mushrooms gathered by anyone but an expert. With regard to household foods, if there is suspicion as to their wholesomeness they are better discarded. Better waste than a serious (occasionally fatal) illness. Tinned foods which have been partly used, and foods cooked and left standing, particularly in hot weather, should be suspect. Frozen poultry should be completely thawed before cooking and cooked food intended for fridge or freezer should be stored as soon as it has cooled to room temperature – not left lying around in a warm state – an ideal incubator for germs. Be very suspicious and careful of any dented or bulging tins. If food poisoning is suspected the remains of the meal should be preserved, and medical help summoned. The patient is best in bed and kept warm.

Fracture. (*Broken Bone*)

The treatment of this falls outside our scope. For those unskilled in first aid the guiding rule with fractures should be to do as little as possible. To move the injured part will often cause further damage. The victim should be made comfortable, kept warm, treated for shock (*see* SHOCK), and the injured part given some support (with as little movement as possible) until medical help arrives.

Freckles.

In women freckles are sometimes a cause of annoyance (though many men find them attractive). There is no effective treatment and if you have the type of skin which pigments in patches instead of all over, as far as possible avoid exposure to the sun.

Frequency of Urination.

Very common. Several causes are dealt with under various illnesses but frequency is sometimes only a symptom of worry, cold, excessive drinking and occasionally follows prolonged love-making. In such instances, the cure is to remove the cause. It does not normally help to reduce fluids except perhaps to abandon late night tea or more especially coffee. Individuals vary greatly in frequency. (*See* CYSTITIS, INSOMNIA, KIDNEY DISEASE, PREGNANCY, PROSTATE, PYELITIS, RETENTION OF URINE.)

Frigidity.

Sexual coldness in the female. It varies from mild indifference to refusal or inability to allow intercourse. The latter type in which penetration is impossible may occur in a woman the first time she has a sex relationship. There may be conditions in the woman or her mate where some physical trouble is the cause; a thick hymen, for example, may need a small operation. These rare instances require prompt advice from the family doctor. They should be curable.

Almost all frigidity is based on fear, guilt feelings or ignorance and happily can usually be conquered with understanding and love – the great aphrodisiac which performs miracles.

All differ in sex needs; some want a lot, others little. Variety in preliminary love play and positions help to prevent boredom. Men often fail to appreciate that most women need to be cuddled and some, intimately kissed, if they are to be turned fully on before intercourse. *For health reasons the importance of careful washing is stressed before any genital kissing.*

Woman's orgasm is not always easy to achieve and this is where knowledge helps. The couple should understand that the clitoris, a tiny "match-stick-head" size "penis" is the nerve centre – indeed the core of a woman's arousal areas (FIG. 8). Successful technique in overcoming frigidity largely depends on knowing this fact. The clitoris lies,

FIG. 8 The female organs

V Vagina B Bladder C Clitoris
W Womb U Urethra opening
L Lips (Labia) H Edge of hymen

protected by what is termed the "hood", where the inner labia (vaginal lips) meet in front. Under stimulation it erects when it may be just large enough to be felt or seen peeping out. It is so sensitive to touch that it must be treated with delicacy. Prolonged tongue-tip caressing here, for some women, by the right man at the right time, can make them wonder how on earth they imagined themselves to be. cold. Not all, but most, men are happy to worship their beloved in this way. The woman must learn to let go, to let her imagination drift and fantasise and abandon herself, rising above thoughts of guilt, for in a loving and caring relationship, there should be none.

In the common intercourse position the woman can make her movements and react against the man's strokes, so that the clitoris should receive the amount of stimulation it needs. Some women can so adjust themselves that they receive the stimulation from the moving penis. Others find this impossible but can adjust their bodies so that the clitoris area is stimulated against the man's pubic area. Certain women like to raise their buttocks with a pillow, while many enjoy the superior position now and again. In the latter the wife is more able to control her stimulation needs. Experimentation is a good word to describe what goes on in the bedrooms of most happy people, while a few less happy couples never get beyond dreaming of it.

There is a group of women who are only able to orgasm in the following way. The woman lies face down, middle raised by a pillow if necessary, legs wide and the man enters the vagina from the back. During his strokes either he or she, using the pad of a clean middle finger, gently but rythmically, stimulates the clitoris. A few couples favour a side by side position, perhaps adjusted with pillows, for this. Such techniques enable millions to enjoy coitus who otherwise could not.

Many couples find love play (and the clitoris, although the centre, is only one of the arousal areas!) sometimes suffices for bodily and spiritual satisfaction instead of slavishly always completing the act. Why not? Heavy petting existed thousands of years before the Pill. The physically handicapped, who have desires like the rest of us, may find this the only way for them, although they can often achieve full intercourse with co-operation and understanding. Love makes nearly everything in marriage possible and love largely consists of giving (and forgiving) as well as receiving.

A few generations ago many women did not enjoy sex because of fears and prejudice. Now most women can achieve some orgasms or discover contentment, release and happiness in the human relationship.

Some older women find sex needs diminish and intercourse painful, while others retain desire into old age. This is no one's fault but for those keen to continue sex chat with your doctor for there are a few medical treatments (other than KY jelly) which may help. In the old, companionship becomes more important and lucky is the woman of whom her man can say "Your body no longer arouses me but my word how up-to-date you have kept your mind".

For any serious difficulty – and they do happen or may develop – visit your doctor.

Frost Bite *and* **Cold Extremities.**

Tissue damage caused by cold. Frost Bite develops in the extremities after exposure. A finger, toe, etc., becomes waxy in appearance and is usually seen in subjects (e.g. mountaineers) who have been exposed to sub-zero temperatures. Treatment is by gradual warming under medical supervision as gangrene (tissue death) is a great risk. The more common painful or numb fingers, especially in the elderly, in everyday cold conditions are best avoided by wearing several layers of warm clothing, avoiding tight garments on the limbs and having regular warm meals. A part which has become numb should be warmed *very* gradually. Here a warm drink is very effective and active rubbing should be avoided. *Trying to help by using hot water can cause excruciating agony, so do not do so.* (*See* REYNAUD'S DISEASE, CHILBLAINS.)

G

Gall Bladder. *(Gall Stones)*

A small hollow pouch attached to the liver. (*See* FIG. 1, *page 31*). It receives bile made by the liver, and pours this into the duodenum where it aids digestion. The gall bladder is sometimes attacked by germs, and becomes inflamed – a condition known as *Cholecystitis*. In some cases, stones form within the gall bladder, and they may cause pain, and can be associated with flatulence and indigestion. Suspected gall stones can usually be seen on X-ray and if present they are often best removed by operation along with the gall bladder. The patient usually recovers well. Gall stones can be dissolved by drugs but this treatment is fairly new; it is possible that stones treated thus may recur.

Ganglion.

A type of cyst in the lining of a tendon often occurring near the wrist. It may cause discomfort but is harmless and often disappears spontaneously in six to twelve months. If it is persistent a minor operation will cure.

Gangrene.

A condition in which a part of the body dies. It is usually due to interference with circulation and may result from a blood clot in the vessel supplying the part (*see* EMBOLISM); or it may be due to progressive narrowing of the blood vessels which keep the part alive. This type of gangrene is not uncommon in the aged, and usually attacks the toe which becomes blackened and shrivels. Elderly people and diabetics should have regular chiropody as small cuts on the feet can precipitate serious trouble.

Gas Poisoning.

Caused by the Carbon Monoxide content of coal gas. England, Wales and Scotland, as well as many other parts of the world are on *Natural Gas* (methane-based) which is not poisonous, but gas poisoning may be possible in other parts of the world where coal gas is still used. (*See* ARTIFICIAL RESPIRATION, ASPHYXIA.)

Gastric Ulcer.

The article on DUODENAL ULCER should be consulted. It is a similar condition arising in the stomach. The pain following meals comes on earlier than in duodenal ulcer – usually in about half an hour, but apart from this the symptoms differ little, and the treatment is similar. Operation is more often advisable for this type of ulcer.

Gastritis.

Inflammation of the stomach, it may follow excessive alcohol or food poisoning. The term is often used for indigestion. (*See* ACIDOSIS *and* DYSPEPSIA.)

General Paralysis of the Insane. *(G.P.I.)* (*See* SYPHILIS)

German Measles. *(Rubella)*

One of the acute infectious childhood illnesses; most children catch it, usually during school years. As with the other illnesses of this nature a second attack is uncommon.

The disease is spread by contact between children, and often occurs in epidemics. The incubation period (the time between contact and the development of symptoms) is generally two to three weeks. The disease often resembles a "cold" at the start, the child having a running nose, eyes, and some fever. There is often enlargement and tenderness in the glands at the back of the neck. The rash usually follows after a short interval starting behind the ears. At first it resembles the rash of measles but is pink rather than dusky consisting of slightly raised round or oval spots. These soon join so there is an almost general redness of the skin. It usually fades after about three days, and may be followed by slight peeling. German measles is not a serious disease and complications are rare.

The patient is infectious for five days after the rash appears. If an expectant mother within the first three months of pregnancy, who has not previously had the disease, comes into contact with it, she should consult a doctor as soon as possible. This is because there is a risk of the unborn baby's development being affected, if the mother contracts the disease.

There is no point in keeping children away from German measles sufferers as it is desirable that they should catch this mild illness and acquire immunity. A vaccine is now available and is offered to all girls in the U.K. at about eleven years. This should ensure immunity during the childbearing years. Adult women who are not immune should contact their G.P. or Local Authority clinic for information. It is imperative that they do not become pregnant within three months of being vaccinated, or be vaccinated while pregnant.

Germs. (*Bacteria, viruses, etc.*)

Name given to small living organisms capable of invading the body and causing disease. Bacteria are measured in microns, each micron being 1/2500th of an inch. There are many types of bacteria, for instance, the staphylococcus which causes boils and the streptococcus which causes tonsillitis. Even smaller are the viruses which cause many illnesses including the common cold and influenza; they can be seen only with a powerful electron microscope.

Giddiness.

The ear is also an organ of balance; there is a special part of the inner ear which helps to maintain our equilibrium. When this is upset we have a sensation of outside objects moving around, and this can occur when the inner ear is over-stimulated by rapid turning (e.g. on a piano stool). Sometimes this part of the ear may be irritated by disease, and true giddiness (vertigo) may result. Tablets such as Stemetil are often helpful. Some patients really mean a feeling of faintness when they talk of giddiness. (*See* FAINT-ING *and* TINNITUS.)

Glands.

There are two different structures in the body referred to as glands. The unqualified term glands usually refers to the lymphatic glands, which are about the size of a pea and are distributed over the body. One of their functions is to filter out the poisons which are liberated when germs invade the body, and when this happens the glands often swell. Thus when germs invade the throat the glands in the neck will often swell up; and with a septic finger, for instance, a swollen gland may often be felt near the elbow.

The other types of gland produce substances which regulate the body's functions. If the gland has a channel or duct down which these substances pass it is known as an exocrine gland. Examples are sweat glands in the skin and the glands producing saliva which reaches the mouth by way of salivary ducts.

If a gland does not have a duct but pours its secretions directly into the bloodstream it is known as a ductless or endocrine gland and the secretion as a HORMONE. Examples are the thyroid, ovary or testicle.

Glandular Fever.

An infective illness, caused by a virus. It commonly attacks children, adolescents and a few adults. The chief symptoms are sore throat and enlargement of the lymphatic glands, often throughout the body (*see* GLANDS). The disease is accompanied by fever, and occasionally a mild rash. The condition often lasts for several weeks, but although very unpleasant in the early days is not usually dangerous, and complications are uncommon. Bedrest is essential during the feverish stage when the spleen may be enlarged and tender. Tiredness can persist up to three months. Antibiotics do not help and treatment is by rest and soluble aspirin.

Glaucoma.

Increased pressure inside the eyeball which if neglected can lead to blindness. It may be heralded by transient mistiness of vision and haloes round lights. Any disturbance of vision should be cause for immediate medical investigation as early glaucoma can usually be contained by appropriate eye drops, before the stage of permanent damage is reached. Pilocarpine has long been of help and new eye drops containing Timolol show great promise. Many are helped by a small operation to aid drainage of fluid from the eye.

Gluten.

The protein in wheat and other grain. Allergy to this produces coeliac disease in which the lining of the intestine becomes damaged so that food cannot be absorbed and malnutrition results. Treatment is by a gluten-free diet. (*See* SPRUE.)

Glycosuria.

The term for sugar in the urine. The usual cause is diabetes.

Goitre.

An enlarged thyroid gland. The thyroid is situated in the front of the neck, either side of the windpipe, and manufactures thyroxine, a hormone, which it pours into the blood. Thyroxine controls the speed at which the body works. With excess the body speeds up – the heart beats faster, weight is lost, etc.; with a lack it slows down. An enlarged thyroid gland may be associated with either too much or too little thyroxine. If there is too much the goitre is said to be "toxic" or the condition may be spoken of as *thyrotoxicosis*. If there is too little the patient is always tired, the body becomes fat and sluggish and the condition is known as *myxoedema*. For a toxic goitre it may be necessary to operate and remove part of the gland, but sometimes operation can be avoided by using drugs which are capable of damping down the action of the thyroid. For the condition of myxoedema, it is necessary to give the patient thyroxine by mouth to restore the normal workings of the body. Sometimes goitre is due to a deficiency of iodine in the diet, and it tends to occur in areas where the water is lacking in iodine. Regular use of iodized salt (made by all leading salt manufacturers) can prevent this type of goitre. (*See* GLANDS, HORMONE.)

Gonorrhoea.

One of the venereal diseases spread by sexual intercourse. It is due to a germ, the gonococcus, which invades the sex organs and sets up inflammation. In the male, symptoms usually commence about four days to a week after intercourse, and there is sometimes some pain on passing water, and may be yellowish discharge from the penis. In the female the symptoms may be delayed and rather indefinite, but pain and some discharge from the vagina are usually present. The pain may seem worse on passing water and women may label this "cystitis". If a woman fears that her "cystitis" could be due to a sexual contact, she should mention this to her doctor so that special tests can be made. Ordinary tests for "cystitis" may miss gonorrhoea. Gonorrhoea can be rapidly cured by antibiotics, but treatment should be started early to ensure the best results.

Neglected gonorrhoea can have serious consequences. In the female it may spread and result in sterility or serious internal disorders, and in the male it may spread to affect the testicles (*see* ORCHITIS). Other unpleasant sequels to neglected gonorrhoea are acute arthritis (*see* ARTHRITIS), and the baby of an untreated mother may develop an infection of the eyes which leads to blindness.

It cannot be too strongly emphasised that if there are *any* symptoms suggestive of gonorrhoea a doctor should be consulted. If the disease is present treatment must be continued until tests show that cure is complete. Doctors at the special V.D. clinics arrange for sexual contacts to be traced and treated. As early symptoms in women may be non-existent a treated man can help his sexual partner (and perhaps many others) by informing her immediately of the risk. Rather a nasty shock now than subsequent abdominal abscesses or sterility later. As always prevention is better than cure. The use of a sheath can prevent infection but is not foolproof. To neglect symptoms or to try to treat oneself by "quack" remedies is to store up trouble for the future – not only for oneself but for others who may become infected. No need for shyness; doctors are not moralists and treatment is confidential. (*See* N.S.U.)

Gout.

A form of painful arthritis caused by crystals of uric acid forming in the joints. The joint most often affected is at the base of the big toe, and the disease manifests itself by recurrent attacks of pain. Other joints can also be involved. Treatment consists briefly in moderation in drinking, reduction of offal in the diet, and in resting the joints during the acute attacks. Tablets can be used to lessen the joint inflammation during such attacks, and allopurinol taken regularly will prevent most recurrences as it reduces the level of uric acid in the body.

Gumma. (*See* SYPHILIS)

H

Haematemesis.

The vomiting of blood. The most common cause is the erosion of a blood vessel in the stomach by an ulcer or by the overfrequent use of insoluble aspirin (*see* GASTRIC *and* DUODENAL ULCER). Often the vomited blood retains its red colour, but sometimes it becomes altered by the gastric juice and assumes a dark brown colour. Anyone with a haematesis should be put to bed and the doctor summoned urgently. Give nothing at all by mouth, but if thirst is complained of the patient may be given a little ice-cold water to sip. Patients should be treated in hospital where transfusion and other treatments can be used if bleeding continues. Sometimes an operation is advisable, but most cases recover without.

Haemophilia.

A rare disease in which the blood fails to clot. Normally if a blood vessel is opened a complicated chemical action starts, which results in a part of the blood gradually becoming solid, and forming a clot. If this did not happen we should be liable to bleed to death from a small cut. In haemophilia a factor necessary for the clotting process is missing. The disease is congenital – i.e. one is born with it. It affects men only, but the condition is "carried" by women who pass it on to their male children. Haemophiliacs can be treated by regular injections of the missing clotting factor.

Haemoptysis.

The medical term for coughing up blood. The blood may be present as streaks in the sputum, is often bright red and may in some cases be frothy. There are many causes including minor chest and throat infections as well as heart disease, lung cancer and blood clot in the lung. Although tuberculosis is now uncommon in the West it is a cause of haemoptysis which is readily treated by modern drugs. Even a tiny haemoptysis should never be ignored. Chest X-rays and other investigations will facilitate prompt treatment.

Haemorrhage.

The general term for bleeding. Internal haemorrhage is when bleeding occurs within the body, external when the blood escapes outside. Most bleeding is due to minor accidents and many people are unduly alarmed by the sight of blood. Recall the experience of thousands of blood donors who give a pint at a time, to see that a quantity of blood may be lost without harmful effects. For bleeding, such as cuts, the best treatment is to apply pressure to the part. This is best done by applying a clean hankie, gauze or cotton wool and bandaging firmly. The bleeding part should be raised – for example if the hand is bleeding the patient should lie on a bed with the hand resting on the head board. The dressing should not be disturbed as this may break up the clot, but if the bleeding continues a further firm bandage may be applied on top of the first. The use of a tourniquet is rarely necessary. Indeed sometimes it is dangerous, for a badly-applied tourniquet may increase bleeding.

Nose bleeds (epistaxis)

The best treatment is to sit over a wash basin with the head slightly forward, the mouth open, a cork between the teeth. The patient should breathe through the mouth and not swallow but allow the blood to run from the mouth. The nose should be squeezed firmly between finger and thumb and a cold pack placed on the bridge of the nose. The reason why nose bleeding often refuses to stop is because patients nearly always swallow the blood which trickles from the back of the nose. Each swallow moves the muscles of the mouth, and causes a tug on the blood vessel which dislodges the clot. By the measure described the vessels remain undisturbed, so that a clot forms and the bleeding stops. Food and drink should be cool for the next twenty-four hours.

Haemorrhoids. (Piles)

Small dilated blood vessels which occur in the region of the anus – the bowel exit, commonly known as *piles*. They are similar to varicose veins. They may cause irritation and some pain, or bleeding from the bowel particularly after the bowels have been opened. Sometimes also a pile "comes down" and protrudes through the anus. Piles may respond to treatment with suppositories and cream e.g. Anusol – twice daily for three weeks or less. The bowel action should be normal – using Isogel and Dorbanex if necessary. Piles can also be treated by injection of a chemical which shrivels them up. It may sometimes be necessary to remove them surgically or treat by dilatation of the anus under anaesthetic. The operation though uncomfortable in the early days is usually successful. Piles sometimes occur in pregnancy, due to increasing pressure caused by the growing child. These usually respond to conservative treatment and often disappear shortly after birth when the abdominal pressure returns to normal. *Haemorrhoids or anal discomfort which fails to respond to ten days' home treatment by suppositories and laxatives should be seen by a doctor.*

Hair. (*See* ALOPECIA *and* BALDNESS)

Halitosis. (*Bad Breath*)
This can occur with local disorders in the gums, teeth, throat or sinuses. It can also occur in distant diseases such as appendicitis, liver disease and diabetic coma as exhaled air contains odorous substances derived from the blood stream. If the cause is removed the trouble should go. Often a person is unduly sensitive about imagined offensiveness of breath. Treatment for anxiety rather than for halitosis may be required.

Hallucination.
A condition in which something which does not exist is perceived. It may refer to any of the senses, so that hallucinations may be seen, felt or heard. They can occur in fever and delirium (*see* DELIRIUM) but are usually a symptom of mental illness e.g. schizophrenia or the result of drugs, e.g. L.S.D. (*see* MENTAL ILLNESS). A hallucination is sometimes confused with a *delusion* which is wrong interpretation of something factual. A patient who looks at a blank wall and sees figures dancing is suffering from a hallucination. A man who hears his wife telephoning the butcher and becomes firmly convinced that she is arranging a meeting with her lover is suffering from a delusion.

Hammer Toe.
A condition in which one of the toes, usually the second, becomes bent down at right angles. Protective felt pads over the toe prevent painful callosities. If pain persists the toe can be straightened by surgery. Often it is associated with bunion and is aggravated by wearing tight shoes. (*See* BURSA).

Hare Lip.
A deep split in the upper lip present at birth and due to a defect in development. It is curable by plastic operations and cosmetic results are excellent. (*See* CLEFT PALATE.)

Hay Fever.

An allergic disease (*see* ALLERGY) in which there is an abnormal sensitivity to pollens. During the summer, trees, flowers and grasses produce thousands of pollen particles which are carried from plant to plant by the air. This pollen is not harmful but in a few who are sensitive it produces irritation of the nose and eyes. The hay fever season usually lasts from May to July, but varies according to which pollen is responsible for the symptoms. Much can be done to help. Tests can be performed by injecting various pollen extracts into the skin to find out which one causes symptoms. Following this injections can be given in which the pollen extract is used in gradually increasing doses. In this way the sufferer can be "desensitized". Antihistamine tablets help as do Rynacrom, Lomusol and Beconase nasal sprays. A long-acting steroid injection is helpful for summer examination candidates who can thus avoid the sedative side-effects of antihistamines; these can cause drivers to fall asleep!

Headache. (*See* MIGRAINE)

A common complaint. Most have a simple explanation; worry, excessive drinking, overwork, hunger, smoking, too little sleep or a minor illness. Most of us suffer an occasional headache and this can usually be relieved by taking two soluble aspirins in a little water. Bathing the forehead with cold water sometimes brings relief but headaches often vanish as mysteriously as they arrive. When headaches become persistent notice must be taken, and some underlying cause sought. Eyestrain (*see* EYE, INFLAMED) should be considered but contrary to popular belief does not often cause headaches. A headache on rising may lead to a suspicion of sinusitis (*see* ANTRUM). ANAEMIA is sometimes a cause, and stress as well as rising blood pressure may induce headaches. The majority of them are not serious, and not an indication of disease of the brain. If, however, headaches occur regularly consult a doctor for advice.

Heart and Heart Disease.

The heart is a specially-adapted muscle, which pumps the blood continuously round the body. The purpose of this is to carry nourishment to the tissues, to take away waste products from the tissues, and, perhaps most important, to distribute oxygen from the air throughout the body. Oxygen makes up about a fifth of the air we breathe, and all living tissues need a constant supply. Air is taken into the lungs where there is a meshwork of tiny blood vessels, and the blood passing through absorbs the oxygen we breathe in. This blood then returns to the heart whence it is distributed via arteries to the body. It returns to the heart after it has lost its oxygen to the tissues, is pumped through the lungs again to collect more oxygen, returns to the heart –

FIG. 9   The contents of the chest
A Trachea, or windpipe   B Bronchi
C Aorta   D Vena Cava   E Heart
F Diaphragm   G Double layer of
pleura covering the lungs   H Ribs
(cross section)

and so on. The heart is a four-chamber pump; two chambers receiving blood (the atria) and two pumping it out (the ventricles). It is also divided into two sides, left and right, each consisting of one atrium and one ventricle.

The heart may be affected in many ways. The muscle may be damaged -- sometimes by the poison from germs, a condition known as *toxic myocarditis*. This may follow various infectious illnesses; but fortunately the damage is often temporary, and the heart muscle recovers. *Rheumatic fever* now fortunately rare in the West, sometimes leaves permanent trouble behind, the heart muscle being weakened and the heart valves damaged. Sometimes, particularly later in life, the muscle is weakened because too little blood reaches the heart itself from the thickened coronary arteries. (*See* ANGINA *and* CORONARY THROMBOSIS.)

In other cases the rhythm of the heart is disturbed. Normally it beats steadily about 70 to 80 times a minute, but sometimes due to disease the pumping action becomes irregular, and less efficient.

The passage of blood through the heart is regulated by valves, which allow the blood to pass in one direction only. Sometimes these are affected by disease, so that they become too narrow, or inefficient, allowing blood to pass in the wrong direction. A common form of valvular disease is aortic stenosis and incompetence. This means that the valve which guards the passage between the left ventricle and the aorta has become thickened and rigid. Nowadays this valve can be successfully replaced by a synthetic model. This is of course a major operation undertaken in specialised centres.

The heart muscle may be strained by having to cope with raised blood pressure but this is slow to develop and the condition is usually recognised before permanent harm is done. Persistent headache, dizziness and shortness of breath might alert one to raised blood pressure and heart strain.

Many drugs help in the treatment of heart disease but one of the most valuable is digoxin, originally obtained from the foxglove. This strengthens the heart beat and slows down erratic rhythms. You can help yourself by keeping your weight down, and giving up smoking. Walking is an excellent exercise and should be increased as far as advised. Worry is the worst enemy. Heart action, like digestion, is involuntary and best left to nature. The heart has a great reserve of power so that even when damaged it is able to cope with basic needs. No activities or interests should be given up unless they provide definite symptoms. Be guided by your doctor. (*See* OEDEMA *and* MURMUR.)

Heartblock.

A condition in which the electrical impulses from atrium to ventricle, are blocked by disease in the "conducting" tissue. Causes are as for heart disease. These impulses regulate the rate of heart beat and if blocked the heart beats too slowly for efficient circulation. Drugs may help but often the insertion of an artificial pacemaker may be necessary.

Heartburn.

A form of indigestion in which burning pain is felt in the centre of the chest. It may be associated with hiatus hernia. (*See* HIATUS HERNIA.)

Hemiplegia.

A condition in which one half of the body becomes paralysed. It is due to some disturbance of the brain, and most commonly follows a stroke. (*See* STROKE.)

Hepatitis.

Inflammation of the liver. The liver may be attacked by viruses either from the blood stream or the digestive tract. When this happens the bile is sometimes unable to escape from the liver, and so passes back into the blood stream causing jaundice. (*See* JAUNDICE, ALCOHOLISM, GALL BLADDER *and* LIVER)

Herbal Remedies.

The beneficial actions of certain herbs have long been known both to physicians and laymen. Even today some of the most important remedies are derived from herbs, e.g. the heart drug digitalis which is obtained from the Foxglove leaf and colchicine used for gout which is obtained from

Autumn crocuses. An interesting new finding is that onions and garlic reduce the levels of cholesterol in our blood and perhaps reduce heart disease. Whilst valuing "natural" medicines we should not disparage new technology which has enabled us to benefit from synthetic medicines.

Hernia. (*Rupture*)

The space within the abdomen is taken up by a number of organs, including the intestines which form a long coiled tube (Fig. 1, *page* 31). The walls of the abdomen, in front, are made of layers of muscle, and if a weakness develops one coil of intestine may push between the muscle layers and come to lie under the skin. It is known as a hernia. The common site is the groin, the weakest part of the abdomen, particularly in men where there is an opening through which the cord passes to the testis. If this becomes stretched a rupture may develop. Ruptures occur in other positions, around the navel or at the site of old operation scars. The best treatment is often an operation. If the space through which the intestine protrudes can be firmly sewn up the rupture will be cured.

It is possible to control a hernia by wearing a truss, or support, which presses on the weak area and should keep the intestine back. A support will not cure and sometimes makes the condition worse, but it should not if the right truss is chosen and it is correctly fitted. For some hernias the flatter type of truss is best. (Made by Sallis Ltd., Nottingham, ND6 ODH.) A hernia may be caused by lifting heavy weights or chronic coughing, etc. Smokers must give up smoking before and after the operation.

Most hernias show as a swelling in the groin which gets larger on coughing, straining, etc. Pain is not marked unless the contents of a hernia become twisted or nipped. The hernia may then be painful and may not reduce back into the abdomen on lying down. Urgent surgical treatment is usually required.

Be guided by your doctor whether a support is needed and if so on what occasions it should be worn. A few find them more suitable worn outside underwear. Nealbourne Ltd., P.O. Box 10, Keighley, West Yorkshire, BD21 4PP, offer a choice of 15 different types of hernia appliances for men and women; mostly very light weight, designed for comfort. Send for brochure. All appliances supplied on 7 days free trial in U.K. Range covers Inguinal, Scrotal and Umbilical Hernias.

If coughing one can, without drawing attention to it, press against the hernia to reduce strain. This can also be done if straining at the toilet. Reasonable exercise helps keep the groin muscles in good condition which may prevent complications. (*See* HIATUS HERNIA.)

Herpes.

A virus causing a group of spots on an area of inflamed skin. The spots (vesicles) have white heads containing fluid. There are two types. Herpes Zoster is the name for shingles (*see* SHINGLES); and another variety Herpes Simplex which develops in areas such as the lips – usually during other illness, e.g. cold. Keep spots dry. They can be dabbed with surgical spirit from time to time and dusted with talcum powder. They usually disappear in days leaving no marks. A variant of Herpes Simplex affects the genital area (*see* SEXUALLY TRANSMITTED DISEASES).

Hiatus Hernia.

An internal hernia where the upper part of the stomach bulges through the opening in the diaphragm intended for the passage of the gullet. The acid stomach contents can thus pass into the sensitive gullet causing pain and inflammation. The condition is aggravated by overweight and tight corsets. Stooping for household tasks and lying flat in bed cause the acid to flow into the gullet. Bending should be done at the knee joint only and several pillows should be used in bed. Antacids and medicines like Asilone and Gaviscon are helpful. The operation to cure is a large one and reserved for severe cases.

Hiccough.

This can be distressing if it refuses to stop. It is usually due to an irritation of the stomach which causes a spasmodic contraction of the breathing muscles resulting in the familiar "hic". One or two glasses of water will often cut an attack short as will firm pinching of the nose for one minute. Recurrent attacks can indicate hiatus hernia (*see* HIATUS HERNIA) or other illness so medical investigation is necessary. Largactil available on prescription will usually stop a severe attack.

Hodgkins Disease.

A form of cancer of the lymph glands (*see* GLANDS). Advances in the last few years mean that this cancer is now readily curable. Symptoms include very enlarged rubbery glands in the neck, armpits or groins. Seek early advice.

Homosexuality.

Sexual attraction towards those of the same sex (usually taken to mean males). Almost everyone is to some extent bi-sexual. If a homosexual is well-adjusted there is no medical indication for treatment. Claims are made that sometimes psychiatric treatment may reverse the condition.

It is normal for some young people to have some homosexual inclinations during their teens and perhaps even into the late twenties. This is a quite usual phase of sexual awakening and they should not make the mistake of thinking that they must be homosexual for life, or allow themselves to be led unnecessarily in this direction. Much active homosexuality is indulged in experimentally and for excitement rather than need.

Some authorities believe that the male homosexual population is a reservoir of V.D. infection. Steady partners are harder to find, so casual sex is more common and indications are that some continue activity before being cleared of the disease, which can also be true in heterosexuality. (*See* LESBIANISM.)

Hormones.

Chemical substances secreted directly into the blood by ductless glands, they affect various body functions. The sex hormones are only one of many types. Where glands are diseased replacement of the appropriate hormone can often be carried out artificially. This is the rationale for hormone replacement therapy at the menopause (*see* MENOPAUSE) when the ovary stops producing oestrogen.

Huntington's Chorea.

A progressive disease of the nervous system which runs in families. Symptoms begin in early middle age and include jerky involuntary movements and intellectual impairment. The Association to combat Huntington's Chorea provides information and help for families of sufferers.

Hydrocoele.

A collection of fluid in the scrotum. It can be present at birth or may develop later in life. Not serious but it can be uncomfortable. Drawing the fluid off via a needle gives temporary relief but the best treatment is by a minor operation.

Hypertension. (*See* BLOOD PRESSURE)

Hypnosis.

Hypnosis is defined as a sleep-like state in which the phenomena of hallucination, memory disturbance and altered behaviour can be induced. However, this relates to the deep state which is less common and for practical purposes hypnosis in most subjects can be regarded as a state of mental and physical relaxation.

The lay concept of hypnosis is usually related to "show-biz" with its dramatic presentation. But what hypnosis is and how it works remains a mystery. Hence methods of induction and clinical uses are still evolving. Traditionally it is used in varied conditions including asthma, migraine and colitis, in the neuroses, in childbirth and gynaecology and in skin diseases and dentistry.

But its most useful applications are in general practice and relate to the many stress reactions people produce to problems of work, finance, housing and marriage and to unpleasant experiences such as a burglary, thunderstorms and examinations, and to assist people to stop smoking and lose weight. Only simple probing of the patient's psyche and past history is necessary in most cases. Simple symptom removal or preferably, symptom tolerance may well be the most useful method in the future. With increasing tolerance and acceptance the psychological overlay or "hang-up" that people get to problems diminishes and this may be followed by a reduction in the patient's stress reaction to their life style. Sometimes hypnosis does not help, other times only to a limited degree, for, like many treatments, it is not magic. But it is worth attempting especially if traditional remedies have failed, for if at worst nothing happens, then at best, the quality of life is enriched. Good results are not uncommon but no guarantee can ever be given.

Hypothermia.

Abnormally low body temperature (*see* TEMPERATURE). Elderly people and babies are less able to maintain normal temperature and in cold weather require more heat than the average. For such people a room temperature of 70°F or 21°C should be ideal – but people differ greatly in needs. Hypothermia often occurs when the elderly patient gets an illness such as a cold or 'flu and cannot get about as usual – keep an eye on your elderly neighbours during the winter.

Hysterectomy.

Operation to remove the womb. The womb is a wonderful container for the developing baby but has no effect on femininity in general. Since one or both ovaries are often retained after this operation the woman need not fear loss of femininity or sudden "menopause" symptoms. If the ovaries must be removed before the menopause because of cysts or other disease, the patient is usually given hormone replacement tablets.

Hysterectomy is usually performed because of heavy, painful periods often due to fibroids. The relief of discarding the source of blood loss usually greatly outweighs the disadvantages of an operation. After six to twelve weeks the woman should feel fully recovered and sexual intercourse can usually be resumed after the first follow-up appointment.

Hysterectomy has no effect on vague ill-health, depression and menopause symptoms like flushing. Women should not imagine that hysterectomy is a cure for all the ills of middle age.

Hysteria.

A nervous disorder in which the sufferer develops impressive symptoms such as total paralysis, total loss of voice, total loss of sensation in the absence of any physical disease. The patient's previous personality has often shown a tendency to exaggerated mood swings. The illness brings some gain e.g. attention or a means of escape from an unpleasant situation but the mental process is not deliberate as in malingering. Hysteria also has a popular meaning when applied to a person who loses control. Following some shock the patient may fling and squirm, go into uncontrollable laughter or tears. A firm hand and sharp words, rather than sympathy, usually produce good results.

Ichthyosis.

A dry and scaly skin condition which sometimes runs in families, ichthyosis is due to a reduction in, or an absence of, the sweat glands which keep the skin moist. It can be alleviated by keeping the skin constantly greased with special ointments such as Unguentum (Merck) or baby oil.

Ileostomy.

Artificial opening of the small intestine (ileum) on to the front abdominal wall. This operation is usually performed where most of the large bowel (colon) is diseased, as in ulcerative colitis, and needs to be removed. Unlike cancer, this condition often occurs in young people so there are many healthy young people around, coping well with this problem. Although the contents of the small bowel are liquid they are odourless so this particular embarrassment is avoided. Disposable polythene bags and attachments make this condition quite easy to manage and much preferable to the miseries of severe colitis. The Ileostomy Association of Great Britain and Ireland exists to give advice and support where necessary. (*See* COLOSTOMY.)

Immunisation. (*Vaccination*).

Protection against disease by the introduction into a susceptible person of a killed or weakened germ in small quantities so as to induce the production of antibodies. Small, modified amounts of the poison normally produced by the germ may be used instead. The antibodies produced are effective against the real germ in spite of having been produced by weaker substances. Doses of vaccine may need to be given more than once in order to achieve full immunity. Boosters are often necessary after a few years. (*See* WHOOPING COUGH, DIPHTHERIA, POLIO *and* TETANUS.)

Impetigo.

An infectious skin disease caused by a germ – the staphylococcus. It usually attacks the face and scalp and is common in children. A small area of skin becomes itchy and inflamed – often near the corner of the mouth – and then begins to weep and form yellowish crusts. If not treated it tends to spread rapidly. Because of this, suspected cases of impetigo are best taken to a doctor as early as possible. It responds to antibiotics. The area affected must be kept dry, and efforts made to prevent the patient scratching for this is one of the chief factors spreading the infection. Bed linen, pillows, handkerchieves and washing materials should be kept strictly separate, and they should be well boiled before being returned to general use.

Impotence.

Inability to perform intercourse by the male. The cause is either bodily or in the mind. Among the usually curable *physical* reasons are: a "stone" pressing on the urethra, interference with the nervous system due to accident or illness. Excessive alcohol or a broken heart can shut down virility until the cause is removed. Prolonged love-making can exhaust the system temporarily. Hormone imbalance may occasionally be the cause.

However, allowing that physical causes can co-exist with psychological, causes in the mind may be responsible for over 95% of impotence, in the sense that when the worries disappear, cure follows. Often the bodily cause arrives *after* the psychological one, because body and mind *affect each other*. Proof is that as soon as the impotent man's confidence is restored, so is his virility.

Sex fears and Taboos go back thousands of years, and some still lurk in the backwaters of our minds. In Victorian times this was perhaps understandable, but since then many pioneering books on sex have been published. Today the enquirer is likely rather to be perplexed by the wide variety of advice available in cheap paperback form. These books reflect the views and prejudices of their authors. Here, however, are a few truths:

Masturbation normally does no harm. Almost every human being has done it, and it is a necessary outlet for those with no partner.

Failure to obtain erection is mainly caused by *fear of failure,* depression or other anxieties. With repeated failure, this fear can feed upon itself. The cure is success, and faith!

Successful erection results when the penis fills with blood due to friction, mental stimulation, or preferably both. Arousal follows kissing, love play, fantasising, or maybe after reading a passionate novel, etc.

Premature ejaculation is a common associated problem. It may even happen before intercourse has started. It is usually caused by a (quite natural) urge to hurry to "get in" before ejaculation. Slow it down and play it cool! If you feel your orgasm coming during foreplay, *stop* and rest. Pause and *breathe deeply* which strengthens control. Finally, enter the vagina at a snail's pace, stopping for a while if you feel orgasm coming too early. A second attempt should be more successful; the point is you cannot damage yourself for Nature does not allow that. If you try too often, the penis refuses to rise until rested, that's all.

Be reassured that (provided there is no extraordinary physical cause) nobody can begin a week virile and end it impotent. Sex problems are not a sign of cowardice. Do not feel guilty. Impotence is not an illness but a symptom and almost always curable.

Love-play can be an occasional alternative to intercourse and sometimes temporarily the only enjoyment following accidents or for the handicapped who have sex needs too. (*See* FRIGIDITY, HOMOSEXUALITY, PROSTATE GLAND.)

Incontinence.

This is when control over the bladder or the bowel is lost. By the age of three bladder control should be established (*see* ENURESIS). The bladder exit is guarded by a muscle; normally it is when we allow this muscle to relax that urine is passed. Incontinence results from many causes. In both sexes it will occur when the nervous control of the bladder is disturbed. Thus a patient may become incontinent after a STROKE when part of the brain is damaged, or an injury to the spine in a road accident. Diseases of the bladder or neighbouring parts may also cause incontinence. Thus it may occur temporarily in CYSTITIS or in prolapse. (*See* PROLAPSE.) Loss of bowel control is also usually due to spinal damage or STROKE. Occasionally in the elderly it is associated with extreme constipation when "spurious" diarrhoea results. Whatever the cause it calls for expert treatment; and anyone who finds difficulty in controlling these functions should consult a doctor. (*See* PARALYSIS, PROSTATE GLAND.)

Indigestion.

This term covers a host of symptoms, and is used when there is any upset in normal digestion. It may be applied to discomfort or pain following meals, heartburn or flatulence. In a medical sense the term has no precise meaning, and does not refer to any definite disease. (*See* ACIDOSIS, DUODENAL ULCER, DYSPEPSIA, FLATULENCE *and* GASTRIC ULCER.)

Infant Feeding *(and Failure to Thrive)*.

In general breast milk (which comes in sterile containers at the right temperature!) is best for feeding babies certainly for the first six to nine months. A few mothers will be unable to do this and can be reassured that carefully prepared bottle feeds provide a good alternative. However, it now seems certain that many mothers who in the past felt obliged to give up breast feeding for reasons like "insufficient milk", engorgement, etc., were probably just lacking the right advice and management at the crucial early stages. In some surveys breast-fed babies have been found to have fewer infections, weight problems or allergies and less coeliac disease, and in later life less heart disease, and less dental decay (their mothers also appear to have less breast cancer). Your health visitor will also be able to advise you before and after the baby arrives.

One of the secrets of success is total demand feeding

without bottle supplements from the earliest hours. This may mean as many as ten feeds a day for the first month reducing in succeeding months. Milk supply depends on frequent sucking, not on some "inherent" factor in the breast. Engorgement is usually due to too infrequent feeds or a rigid schedule. You should feed your baby when he cries, if your breasts feel full, whenever "you feel like it" and if he goes for as long as four hours without a feed. It is possible to underfeed a young baby who may sleep for long periods giving the illusion of contentment. Sadly, this can lead to an apparently "contented" baby being severely undernourished. *Few babies under three months can manage on less than five daily feeds.*

The bottle-fed baby has a minor advantage as his feeds can be measured. As a rough guide a young baby needs $2\frac{1}{2}$ozs milk per pound of body weight daily. Thus after the first week, a seven pound baby needs $17\frac{1}{2}$ozs milk divided into five or six feeds i.e. approximately 3oz at a time. Baby will take different amounts at different times but this gives some idea.

Babies gain roughly 4 to 7oz of weight weekly in the early months. If they *consistently* fail to do so it usually means something is wrong and advice from health visitor or doctor is needed. Apart from the usual cause, which is a feeding problem, the others are infection, particularly in the waterworks and, rarely, congenital defects such as heart disease.

Solid food such as cereal should not be offered until four months at the earliest. A proprietary brand of rice suitable for infants is one of the least stodgy solids to begin with. One teaspoon with one of the daily feeds is enough to start and you can gradually build up over the subsequent months. Sieved vegetables and fruit and finally meat meals can be introduced slowly. Baby will probably have fads and fancies but do not worry about it as milk supplemented by vitamin drops is his most important food for the first nine or ten months. When teething begins around six months he will, of course, want to bite on something a little harder such as a rusk; but he is unlikely to eat more than half of it. The nutritional value of a rusk is similar to cereal.

A relaxed mother is likely to have less problems with

feeds than a mother who is tense, so she should aim to put aside a little time daily for her own interests and relaxation.

Infantile Paralysis. (*See* POLIOMYELITIS)

Infection.

This occurs when the body is invaded by germs. It may be local as in a boil, or a generalised infection like measles. A disease is *infectious* when the germs can be spread indirectly from person to person. Thus "colds" are infectious, being spread by coughing and sneezing. Some diseases are spread by direct contact and these are *contagious*. An example is venereal disease in which the germs are normally spread only by sexual contact with a diseased person.

Infertility.

Properly thought of as sub-fertility for few people are totally infertile. Pregnancy occurs when an egg (released monthly from the woman's ovaries) passes into the Fallopian tube and is fertilised by a male sperm. This fertilised egg continues along the tube to the womb where it embeds in the soft lining. This process requires that all is well with the ovaries, tubes, uterus, uterus lining, cervix and vagina. The ovary is influenced by the pituitary gland below the brain and is subject to nervous factors.

In the man the mechanism of erection and ejaculation must operate, the production of sperms by the testicle must be satisfactory in quality and quantity and there must be an unblocked passage along the male tube (vas) along to the storage pouch (seminal vesicle) and then on into the passage through the penis. Fluid from the prostate gland is also added to the semen at ejaculation. Most couples are probably infertile at some time after a bout of influenza or a period of exhaustion.

The ovum is usually released about day 14 of the average twenty-eight day period cycle (counting the first day of a period as day one). Both egg and sperm have a limited life – not more than one to two days – so only intercourse on day 13 to 16 approximately is liable to result in pregnancy (this cannot be relied on for contraception – *see* CONTRACEPTION).

If after six months to a year of being in good health and having had intercourse at least three times a week especially at mid-cycle, there is still no sign of a baby it is worth seeing a doctor to see if there is some easily remedied cause. One assumes that this healthy young couple are taking a balanced diet, plenty of protein, fibre foods and vitamins, also exercise and joy in each other's company. Female orgasm does seem to help "suck in" sperms and this should be occurring at least on some occasions but is not essential. (*See* FRIGIDITY.)

Sometimes the reassurance of the feeling that "something is being done" provides the necessary relaxation and it is common to find the woman is pregnant by the time her specialist appointment comes along!

While waiting for a gynaecological appointment a woman can obtain a good idea of whether or not she is ovulating (releasing an egg) regularly by recording her oral, early morning temperature before rising or having any drink. This should be charted against date and the day of her period cycle. A tiny fall followed immediately by a half degree F ($\frac{1}{4}°$C) rise which continues until the end of the cycle indicates ovulation. If this is occurring regularly there is no problem with ovulation. An erratic chart and infrequent or scanty periods usually mean that eggs are not being released regularly. Such a patient may benefit from clomiphene tablets to regularise ovulation. These are not to be confused with the hormone injections which can produce multiple births. These are necessary only for a very few patients who fully understand the risks and wish to take their chance.

Sometimes minor abnormalities such as small fibroids, an erosion (ulcer on the neck of the womb) or backward tilting of the womb are found and these can often be corrected surgically with good results. Blocked tubes due either to advanced appendicitis, tuberculosis or venereal disease are a more difficult problem. The promiscuous nineteen year old rarely spares a thought for her future sorry state at 30+ with blocked tubes and the adoption waiting lists closed. Operations to unblock them are not over-successful although Fallopian tube transplants are being tried. Sometimes where tubes are blocked by thread-

-like adhesions they can be cleared by insufflation with carbon dioxide (during a period).

Test Tube Baby

The test tube baby technique as used in the U.K. was devised to overcome a problem of totally blocked tubes due to appendicitis. A method was devised for estimating exactly the time of ovulation and an egg was removed from the ovary at this point. The minor operation done under a general anaesthetic was performed through a type of tele- scope (the laparoscope) so that a minute incision only was necessary. The egg was mixed with the husband's fresh semen in a tube and was re-implanted into the womb lining at night (apparently the best time for a "take"). Thereafter pregnancy continued in the normal way. This is the most *extreme* form of A.I.H. (Artificial Insemination Husband).

In less extreme cases the gynaecologist can place the husband's semen directly in the neck of the womb, via a syringe, where there is some problem like unusual position of cervix, a potency problem, etc. Where there is a low sperm count several specimens of the husband's semen can be centrifuged and a more concentrated liquid inserted.

To consider the male aspect a little more. A simple semen test arranged by the family doctor may show any- thing from a satisfactory vigorous number of sperms to fewer sperms or some condition needing treatment. Some- times even the healthy ones become sluggish on contact with the mucus contained in the woman's cervix. This can be confirmed by a test on the woman some hours after intercourse. Further hormone tablets for the woman usu- ally help this as does A.I.H. Nowadays the sperm count can often be improved by treatment such as hormone tablets. Even complete absence of sperm in the seminal fluid may simply mean a blockage somewhere along the sperm col- lecting tubes whilst sperm production by the testicle is normal; this may be amenable to plastic surgery. Some- times the position corrects itself.

If nothing further can be done to help the man's prob- lems whereas his wife has normal fertility the question of A.I.D. (Artificial Insemination Donor) arises. Often the couple wish to have a child that is at least part their own flesh and blood and if both parties are in agreement the technique is similar to that of A.I.H. The voluntary donor is always young and healthy, often a medical student. Total secrecy is maintained as to his identity.

Here are some small tips which may help a couple who do not so far feel that medical help is necessary. Since in intercourse the semen has to travel along the cervical canal, through the uterus and up the fallopian tubes, it may help if the woman remains on her back with hips raised on a pillow for twenty minutes after intercourse; even better if the couple remain in this position together, without moving much.

If the uterus is tilted backwards the sperms tend to be deposited behind the cervix rather than onto it. Intercourse in which the man enters from behind helps to place the semen in the right place. It is worth trying this position several times even if you are not sure in which position your womb is lying.

Abstention from intercourse for a few days increases the sperm count but this should not be taken to extremes. A three day abstention before intercourse at estimated ovulation time is all that is necessary. Douching before intercourse with half a teaspoon bicarbonate to a half pint of warm water has been found helpful by some.

Often after many tests the specialists tell you that they cannot find any reason why you should not conceive. Although in these circumstances a baby may arrive seven to ten years or more after your anxieties first began it is possibly wise to approach the adoption agencies. Although white, healthy babies under a year are in short supply there are babies of mixed race, and some with handicaps, and some older children available. This will take your mind off the obsessional concentration on period cycles, etc., and of course everyone knows how often a woman becomes pregnant shortly after adopting a baby.

Inflammation.

The reaction of a body tissue to injury – provided the injury is not sufficient to kill the part. It does not matter much what form the injury takes: traumas, heat, cold or infection. The part becomes swollen and red because the small blood vessels are widely opened; for the same reason it is usually painful because nerve endings are irritated. An example is a boil which shows the characteristic signs of inflammation, being swollen, red, hot, and painful.

Influenza.

An acute generalised infection which occurs in epidemics. Several different types of virus cause slightly different kinds of 'flu. The disease usually starts with a fever and aches and pains in limbs, back and head. The patient feels unwell and alternately hot and shivery. There may be watering of eyes and nose followed by a sore throat and irritating cough. Later on sickness may be a feature and in this case the illness is often spoken of as "gastric flu". It is not usually serious, though there have been severe epidemics. The temperature settles down usually within a week, and the patient gradually returns to health. It is chiefly dangerous because it lowers the body's defences and may be followed by complications like pneumonia. It is not a condition to neglect, and the patient should remain in bed until the temperature is normal for 24 hours. Depression is common following influenza and convalescence should not be hurried.

There is at present no specific treatment for influenza. Antibiotics are not a cure; they are only of use for complications like bronchitis. Vaccines have been developed for many strains of influenza; if given in October they can be effective for the winter. Alas, the influenza virus frequently changes and becomes resistant to the vaccines. Protection against one epidemic will not necessarily protect against the next.

Ingrowing Toe Nail.

This is common. The surrounding skin fold becomes raised at the edge so the nail instead of growing over grows *into* it causing pain. The skin fold often becomes infected and may discharge pus. It may be due to tight shoes, particularly in childhood. To prevent, care should be given to fitting shoes especially in the young (*see also* BURSA). The nails should be cut straight across, *not into an oval*, and the services of a chiropodist are often worthwhile. For severe cases it is sometimes necessary to have a small operation.

Insanity. (*See* MENTAL ILLNESS)

Insomnia.
Inability to sleep is a tiring condition. It becomes common with age. Those troubled should read the section on Sleep, page 12. If that does not cure consult a doctor. Often simple remedies such as covering the eyes over to keep out the light or if noise prevents sleep, several types of earplugs may be helpful. A hot bottle to cold feet can do the trick. Thinking happy thoughts, a sexless cuddle of one's mate or intercourse can work but possibly a holiday, away from it all, is best. Some people find sitting up supported by pillows or using an extra pillow helps unless they happen to have any neck trouble. A well-made bed is important; if the sheet is not wrapped to cover the blankets, the latter can tickle the face and prevent sleep.

Insulin.
A hormone produced by the pancreas which controls the rate the body burns up sugar and starchy food. (*See* DIABETES, GLANDS, HORMONES.)

Intussusception.
Where one part of the intestine telescopes into another. Sufferers are usually male babies between six and twelve months old who suffer severe colic, accompanied by screaming and drawing up of the knees. Often there is sickness, and in some a little dark red blood is passed from the bowels. The condition calls for urgent treatment. An operation is usually required.

Iritis.
A serious but readily treated cause of a red painful eye. It is due to inflammation of the iris (coloured part of the eye which acts as a diaphragm to light). The pupil is usually small and the iris seems cloudy in this condition. Urgent treatment is required. Drops may suffice but corrective

steroid injections into the eye are usually needed. (*See* EYE, EYESIGHT.)

Itch. (*See* SCABIES)

Caused by mild irritation of the skin, it is a common symptom of many skin diseases. Scratching cures an itch temporarily by swamping the messages which travel up the nerves by more powerful ones; but in the long run it often makes it worse by increasing the irritation. For a mild itchiness calamine lotion is often effective. If it is not, see your doctor as there is possibly a skin condition which can be treated.

J

Jaundice.

One function of the liver (*see* LIVER) is to make bile, a dark green liquid stored beneath the liver in a pouch known as the GALL BLADDER. It pours into the intestine where it helps the digestion of fats. If the bile cannot escape into the bowel it is forced back into the liver and enters the blood stream. The skin and the whites of the eyes then become coloured yellow (the former not visible in the yellow or coloured races). This is *jaundice*. Whatever the cause the sufferer usually feels *extremely* ill with vomiting, no appetite and abdominal pain. There are many causes.

(1) Jaundice can occur in new born infants due to the immaturity of the liver which cannot quite cope with its various functions. This type usually clears within days but can be treated by ultraviolet ray therapy if necessary. Where there is incompatability between the parents' blood groups, especially of the rhesus factor (*see* RHESUS), the jaundice may be more serious. If ultraviolet ray treatment is not effective, exchange blood transfusions may be needed.

(2) Infectious hepatitis (*see* HEPATITIS) – the liver may be attacked by a virus which causes inflammation, damaging liver cells and blocking the ducts which carry the bile. Other germs and viruses can also attack the liver. Sometimes GLANDULAR FEVER is complicated by jaundice.

(3) Mechanical blockage of the bile ducts always leads to jaundice. Sometimes stones develop in the gall bladder and one of these may obstruct the duct which takes bile into the intestine. This duct may also be blocked by enlarged lymph glands or by a tumour.

(4) Excessive destruction of red blood cells which occurs in some types of anaemia can lead to jaundice.

(5) Damage to liver cells by poisons can cause jaundice. Such poisons include carbon tetrachloride used in dry cleaning, some of the poisonous toadstools and excessive consumption of alcohol. (*See* ALCOHOLISM.)

All types of jaundice need urgent medical attention. In young people the commonest form is infectious hepatitis. It is spread by infected food and drink and possibly by breathing virus-contaminated air. A similar but much more serious form of hepatitis, known as serum hepatitis is acquired directly from infected blood and can be transmitted by dirty syringes and occasionally by blood transfusion (rarely in the U.K.). This is why a person with a past history of jaundice can never be a blood donor. It is possible to be a carrier of the disease for many years while feeling perfectly well. Drug addicts dependent on shots of heroin from dirty syringes risk serum hepatitis and there is evidence that the disease can be transmitted by sexual intercourse among casual contacts who may be carriers, commonly found among homosexuals.

Treatment of infectious hepatitis consists of bed rest, low fat diet and complete abstinence from alcohol. Alcohol should not be taken for at least six months, even though the symptoms may have cleared in the first weeks. Relapse of jaundice can occur if this rule is not obeyed. Cases of serum hepatitis may need to be admitted to specialist hospital units for intensive treatment.

K

Kidney Diseases.

The kidneys are two organs at the back of the abdominal cavity. They filter the blood continually passing through them, and remove waste products which are then disposed of in the urine. The kidneys may be the seat of acute inflammation known as *nephritis*. It is due to a delayed response of the body to the streptococcus germ which causes sore throats and tonsillitis. The normal defensive action against the germ is "overdone" and actually causes damage elsewhere in the body – sometimes the kidneys – some six weeks after the original infection. A change for the better in the nature of the streptococcus germ plus the use of penicillin in the treatment of tonsillitis has greatly reduced this illness. Symptoms are pain in the loins, fever and the dark red urine due to the presence of blood. There may also be swelling beneath the eyes and the lower parts of the body due to water in the tissues (*see* OEDEMA). Urgent medical treatment is needed.

Sometimes infection ascends the kidney tubes from the bladder leading to pyelonephritis. In this there is usually a high temperature, pain in the loins, and great frequency in passing water. This infection needs urgent investigation and treatment with antibiotics.

In some patients severe disease may result in failure of the kidney to remove poisonous waste products from the blood. (*See* URAEMIA.) Modern treatments have revolutionised the outlook for these people. Artificial kidney machines often installed in the patient's own home can replace the work of the patient's own kidneys by filtering the blood. Sufferers are usually "plugged in" three nights a week and they and their families become adept at handling the apparently complicated machinery. Many are helped by kidney transplants when a suitable "matching" donor kidney is available. Transplant patients need continual treatment with drugs to prevent their rejecting the new kidney, but they usually feel remarkably well.

We can all help such patients by agreeing to make our kidneys available for transplant after our death. Kidney donor cards for signature by donor and next-of-kin are available in doctor's surgeries, hospital out-patients departments and Local Authority Clinics.

Sometimes stones develop in the kidney and escape causing pain and bleeding as they pass down the duct (or ureter) from the kidney to the bladder. Medical investigation is necessary. (*See* CALCULUS *and* RENAL COLIC.)

Knock-Knee.

A condition in which the ankles are some distance apart when the knees are placed together. This is commonly seen in healthy young children and will correct spontaneously in 99% of cases. Provided that the distance between the ankles is not greater than 10 cms (4 ins) in a four year old the parents can be reassured that the condition should be correct without treatment. In the few persistent cases, orthopaedic stapling or operation near maturity when the bones are matured give good results.

Bow legs (which curve outwards below the knee, and then back in again) in British children are rarely due to dietary deficiency and again are normal in many toddlers who grow out of the condition by the age of four. Rickets due to inadequate vitamin D (see PAGE 10) may be a cause in Asian and other children. Treatment here is by extra vitamin D (cod liver oil, ABIDEC drops), calcium (syrup of calcium gluconate) and orthopaedic maneouvres. In later life bone disease such as Paget can cause bowing of the legs.

L

Labia.

Derived from Latin; it means lips. It is the name for the double folds of skin which form part of the external female organs. There are two labia, an inner and outer on each side of the mid-line. Close to the inner pair are a number of small glands (see BARTHOLIN'S GLANDS) whose function is to lubricate the part during sexual intercourse.

Labour. (*See* BIRTH)

Laryngitis.

The larynx (voice box) lies in the neck at the top of the windpipe, below the throat. It is liable to become inflamed in any infection of the respiratory (breathing) organs, and laryngitis may follow or accompany such conditions as a "cold" or bronchitis. It often starts with "tickling" low in the throat followed by a cough, which becomes painful. If the attack is severe the larynx cannot function properly so that the voice becomes husky, sometimes only a whisper. The condition usually clears in about a week or can be relieved by inhaling steam to which soothing medicaments such as Friars' Balsam (one teaspoon to a pint) have been added. Honey and lemon preparations are soothing but if the condition is not improving antibiotics from your doctor may help.

Lesbianism. (*See* HOMOSEXUALITY)

Sexual attraction between two women; possibly more common than is thought, but serious instances probably rare – lesbians usually being bi-sexual.

Leucorrhoea.

The name given to slight excess of the *normal* creamy white discharge from the vagina. There is normally more discharge at puberty, when the sexual functions are becoming established, also for a few days before each period, and often during pregnancy. This type of discharge is never irritant or offensive. Any discharge which seems more than normal leucorrhoea, is offensive, or which causes soreness, itching or irritation must be investigated. Your doctor is used to such matters and it is better to have the condition put right early. (*See* GONORRHOEA, N.S.U., VAGINITIS.)

Leukaemia.

The name given to a disease in which the white cells or corpuscles in the blood multiply. The function of white cells is chiefly to deal with invading germs, and their number is normally relatively low compared to red cells. The condition of *leukaemia* may be regarded as a form of cancer in which the white cells continue to multiply indiscriminately. There are many types of leukaemia. The white cells can be broadly divided into two categories known as lymphocytes and myelocytes.

Acute leukaemia of the lymphocytes occurs in young children and is thus one of the most distressing forms of cancer. Modern methods of treatment are however giving promising results. Treatment with special drugs and radiation can keep the disease suppressed in over half the patients treated and some cases are cured. The treatment is complicated and must be given in specialist centres. Symptoms at the onset are vague but include persistent tiredness and listlessness. Usually there is a simple explanation like the common childhood infections or mild anaemia but if the parents are worried a simple blood test will establish the facts.

Unfortunately the types of *acute* leukaemia which occur in young adults are proving difficult to cure as yet. In older people the *chronic* leukaemias can be treated with good results in most cases. Such patients can often lead normal lives for twenty to thirty years after the original diagnosis.

FIG. 10   Lice

1   Body louse   2   Pubic louse   3   Nit

Lice.

Small animal parasites, the size of a match head. They live on the human body and usually inhabit hairy regions, cementing their eggs, or nits, to a hair after they are laid. There are three families; the head louse, the body louse, and the pubic louse. *Pediculosis* is the medical term for infestation by lice. The condition is contagious as lice spread from one person to another. Infection by body lice is encouraged by lack of personal cleanliness. Lice flourish when washing becomes difficult, as for instance, in fighting soldiers. The louse feeds on blood from its host, and the bites cause irritation. Scratching may introduce germs so that infected spots and small boils develop. A grave consequence is the spreading of a disease known as *Typhus,* a serious illness caused by a small germ which, apart from attacking a man, can live in the body of the louse. Infected lice may spread from person to person, carrying the disease with them.

Pubic lice are commonly transmitted by sexual activity and other tests for venereal disease should always be carried out where pubic "crabs" are found.

Unlike the body lice *head* lice are no respectors of personal cleanliness and will spread rapidly round a clean room of clean school children if one child has them. The sharing of combs, head gear and towels is to be discouraged.

Treatment of head and pubic lice is by malathion liquid left on for thirty minutes, then shampooed off. Body lice can be treated by quellada lotion applied to whole body except head and left on for 24 hours before washing off. The hair is combed with a fine-tooth comb before drying to remove nits. Treatment can be repeated in 48 hours.

Limp.

In general a limp is nature's way of protecting an injured limb from undue strain and of indicating a disorder. An injury to a limb is bound to produce some degree of limp for a time.

However, a limp occurring without a preceding injury in a child or teenager between the ages of five and eighteen years should never be ignored as there are two important considerations which may be present and which should be caught in the early stages. Associated pain may be in the thigh, groin or even the *knee*. In one condition the growing part of the top of the thigh bone slips out of place *(slipped epiphysis)* and if not corrected leads to permanent limp and later arthritis. In the other disorder the top of the thigh bone tends to become flattened and again the later development of arthritis is likely if the condition is neglected.

Babies at the crawling stage or who have just begun to walk need early medical advice if they consistently refuse to bear any weight or use an arm or leg. Whilst older children may occasionally limp in order to get attention a limp in a toddler always means damage, possibly a fracture. Some babies are born with dislocated hips and routine examination in the first weeks of life usually spots these. Treatment is by plaster or splinting and results are good. Unfortunately a few are not found so early. A limp or discrepancy in thigh length in newly walking babies demands urgent investigation.

Lipoma.

The name given to a fatty tumour. The body is normally covered by a layer of fat beneath the skin, and sometimes, instead of being distributed evenly, the fat in one place forms into a soft, painless lump – about the size of an egg, beneath the skin. The tumours are harmless, but sometimes unsightly. They can easily be removed by operation.

Liver.

A large organ in the upper right side of the abdominal cavity (Fig. 1, *page 31*); it serves important functions. The blood from the digestive tract passes through the liver before it returns to general circulation. A lot of the nourishment from food is altered by the liver to make it suitable for body use. Some food, particularly sugar, is stored in the liver so that it can be used later if the body requires it. The liver also removes worn-out blood corpuscles from the circulation and uses the red pigment (haemoglobin) from the red blood cells in the manufacture of the bile. This bile is stored in the GALL BLADDER and then poured into the intestine where it helps the digestion of fats. Inflammation of the liver is known as hepatitis (*see* HEPATITIS *and* JAUNDICE), and sometimes the cells degenerate so that the liver becomes scarred and can no longer carry out its functions properly a condition known as *cirrhosis of the liver*. Although there are other causes, excessive alcohol is one important cause of cirrhosis. You do not have to be an alcoholic to get cirrhosis; regular social drinking of more than three pints of beer daily can cause damage. (*See* ALCOHOLISM.)

Lobar Pneumonia. (*See* PNEUMONIA)

Lumbago. (*See* BACKACHE)

Lupus Vulgaris.

A rare form of skin tuberculosis occasionally seen in tropical areas, readily treated with modern anti-tuberculous drugs.

Lymphadenoma. (*See* HODGKINS DISEASE)

M

M and B. (*See* SULPHONAMIDES)

Malaria.

One of the commonest illnesses in the world, it is spread by the Anopheles mosquito. The tiny parasite is transferred by a bite to human red blood cells. Once established in the human blood it causes high fever, and prostrating illness which tends to recur. The Department of Health, of London, can advise you if your destination requires malaria protection. Anyone travelling to sub-tropical or tropical areas should take precautionary tablets such as Chloroquine 400 mgms weekly starting before they travel and for six weeks after returning. If the disease develops urgent medical attention is required.

Mania and Hypomania. (*See* MENTAL ILLNESS)

Terms covering abnormal states of excitement which affect people who are subject to mood swings and it may be difficult to decide if there is illness or merely great energy. Mild cases (hypomania) appear restless, talkative and over-excited or may seem euphoric. Like all mental illnesses, mania can arise from prolonged stress. Manics can plunge into depression (*see* DEPRESSION) but the outlook is usually very good with prompt treatment.

It may be difficult for the patient with early hypomania to be persuaded to accept help as the euphoria leads him to believe he is healthy. Where there is a past history one must watch for danger signs as the patient rarely complains. Advanced symptoms include euphoric ideas, etc., and sufferers become increasingly active driving themselves to exhaustion. The immediate essential is to control the exhausting, useless activity which can become frightening. A doctor will decide whether hospital treatment is indicated but if there is fear that the patient might harm himself or others in the interim, police aid must also be summoned.

After the acute stage, the patient should respond to medicines such as lithium and to psychological explanations including commonsense discussion of the factors which have upset him. (*See* MENTAL ILLNESS.)

Mastitis.

Inflammation of the breast which can lead to abscesses (*see* BREAST). The term is now often used to mean the discomfort which some women experience in the breast each month shortly before the period. It is due to fluid retention in the breasts and increase in glandular tissue which can be felt as general "lumpiness" (not a single lump which requires urgent investigation). The monthly variation in female hormones accounts for these changes and some women seem more prone to this than others. Symptoms can be eased by diuretics (tablets to eliminate fluid). If you are doubtful about nodules in the breast do check with your doctor. They may well be due to this harmless condition but medical assessment is necessary. (*See* PREMENSTRUAL TENSION.)

Mastoid.

The mastoid process is a projection from the bones of the skull behind the ear (Fig. 6, *page* 87). In common with several skull bones it is hollow (*see* ANTRUM), and contains small spaces filled with air. These spaces communicate with the inside of the ear, so if there is a neglected infection of the middle ear the mastoid may become involved. The condition, now rare, is known as *mastoiditis*. The pus from the infection cannot easily escape and may, if left, work inwards until it causes a brain abscess. Mastoiditis is usually accompanied by discharge from the ear, and the bone behind becomes painful. There is often a high temperature, and severe headache. Modern drugs, such as penicillin, usually cure but occasionally an operation is necessary to allow the pus to escape. Prompt treatment of earache should eliminate this condition.

Masturbation.

Self-gratification of the sex urge. In both sexes there is a strong instinct towards sexual union, but under civilised conditions this must be controlled. Marriage offers an outlet for the sex drive, but some people marry late or remain single. With them the urge must either be inhibited or gratified outside marriage or by self-relief. The last, especially among the young of both sexes, is common, normally harmless and preferable to promiscuity with its risks of illegitimate pregnancy, broken hearts or venereal disease.

Abnormal sperms are common after abstinence so regular release seems to have some beneficial effect on fertility. (*See* FRIGIDITY *and* IMPOTENCE.)

Measles.

An infectious disease of childhood caused by a virus. The disease usually occurs in epidemics and commonly affects children, though older people who have escaped may develop it. A second attack is rare. The incubation period, i.e. the interval between "catching" the germ and developing the disease, is usually about ten days. The early symptoms resemble a severe "cold" and usually come on suddenly with shivering, headache, running and redness at the eyes and nose. A troublesome barking cough is a marked feature and the child is often brought to the doctor for "chestiness". The temperature rises gradually until the rash develops. This is usually on the fourth day, though before the spots develop on the skin they can be seen, often on the inside of the cheeks, as small red spots with a bluish-white centre.

The rash proper starts as small, dusky red slightly raised spots which soon run together, giving the skin a blotchy appearance. The spots appear behind the ears, then on the face, and later spread over the body. After about three days the rash usually begins to fade, the temperature settles, and the patient begins to recover. Measles is in fact an acute bronchitis with rash thrown in and mother will find she is looking after a very chesty child for a few days. Linctuses such as phensedyl are helpful and doctors may recommend antibiotics at the start of an attack to prevent complications.

The child needs rest and quiet, plenty of fluids and soluble aspirin if he is achey or feverish. Since the disease lowers resistance, it may be followed by complications such as inflammation of the ears, and occasionally pneumonia. The patient may be given a full diet once the appetite returns, and is best in bed for a few days until the temperature has returned to normal.

Children are now offered inoculation against measles in their second year of life so this distressing disease should not occur. Mothers fearing any brain damage from the vaccine should remember that brain inflammation is more likely from the disease itself.

Melaena.

When blood escapes into the upper part of the digestive tract it becomes altered by the digestive juices, and is changed from red into a black, tarry semi-solid mass. The passage of this altered blood from the bowels is known as *melaena*. There are a number of causes. Bleeding from a gastric or duodenal ulcer may cause blood to pass into the intestines instead of being brought up (*see* HAEMATEMESIS). Other diseases of the stomach and small bowel may also result in bleeding and melaena. Melaena is an indication of serious illness and prompt medical advice is needed.

Melanoma.

A tumour of the skin which may be brown or black due to the pigment melanin. Malignant change may occur in the pigment cells and this type of cancer is commoner in fair-skinned people over-exposed to sunlight. If a mole or freckle becomes larger, bleeds, itches or becomes sore consult your doctor since this type of skin tumour is often curable by a simple operation but only when caught early.

Meningitis.

The meninges are three layers of membrane which provide covering for the nervous tissue in the brain and spine. *Meningitis* is an inflammation of the meninges and *always needs urgent medical attention*. It may be caused by germs which attack the nervous system, and one in particular, the meningococcus was once responsible for epidemics. The onset in this type is sudden, and the most prominent symptom is very serious headache with stiffness of the neck. There is always fever, prostration and sometimes vomiting. This form of meningitis responds to antibiotics if diagnosed and treated early.

Another form of meningitis, now rare in the U.K., is caused by infection with the tubercle bacillus. The discovery of "Streptomycin" and other antibiotics effective against the tubercle bacillus has greatly improved the outlook. The most common form of meningitis today is viral or aseptic meningitis. Symptoms are similar to meningococcal meningitis but the disease runs a milder course. Lumbar puncture and examination of the spinal fluid confirm the diagnosis. Treatment is usually by rest and analgesics and occasionally steroids in the form A.C.T.H. Nowadays complete recovery from viral meningitis is usual.

Menopause.

Between 45 and 53 a woman normally becomes incapable of childbearing. Sometimes the periods stop suddenly, but in some they become scanty or irregular before they finally cease. Many important bodily functions are controlled by various glands (including the ovaries) which pour hormones into the blood stream. These glands are under control of a "master" gland, the pituitary, connected with the brain. At the menopause the ovaries gradually cease to function, and this often upsets the balance between the pituitary and other glands, so that it takes time for the body to settle down to normal. Various unpleasant symptoms may result. Hot flushes, due to excess of one particular hormone, are often troublesome. There may be some weight gain although this is often due to decreased physical activity and enjoyment of sweet food rather than to true glandular effects. Minor mental upsets may occur. Depression is common at the menopause and if it does not seem to improve with plenty of company and activity see your doctor in case depression treatment is indicated. Migraines may also begin at this time (see MIGRAINE) but fortunately there are many forms of help for this.

By the menopause the woman's family has often grown up and left home and she may feel that she is leading a rather empty life. Now is the time to think of taking up a job, outdoor sport, voluntary work – anything to take your mind off yourself and return to happier living for you may well have half your life to live.

At a more serious physical level there is loss of calcium from the bones in menopausal women; think how common wrist fractures are in older women. Extra calcium does not seem to help although it may reduce pain associated with bone thinning.

A few, but not all, women lose interest in sex at the menopause; if people want their sex life to continue longer it seems that those who retain the greatest interest in the subject find that helps greatly. Problems may be due partly to vaginal dryness (easily put right by KY Jelly). The vaginal lining also becomes more delicate and easily inflamed after the menopause. Some women may benefit from the *occasional* use of oestrogen cream to cope with this.

Oral oestrogen replacement (H.R.T.) may help some if not all of the symptoms mentioned. The oestrogens must be given cyclically as in a normal period cycle and they must be combined with a progestogen which allows a regular monthly "period" to shed any tissue which may have been building up in the uterus. Some women are reluctant to return to a monthly "period"; others with a strong family history of heart or artery disease or who have had a deep vein thrombosis themselves or who have marked varicose veins would be ill advised to take oestrogens.

However, for some with crippling hot flushes, moodiness and weight fluctuations oestrogen replacement has given worthwhile improvement. It would be of great benefit if it were shown that calcium was retained in bones in women on H.R.T. but as yet this is not definitely proved. If you are having *distressing* symptoms with the menopause see your doctor who should be able to help one or other way.

Menorrhagia.

The term for heavy periods in women – often known as *flooding*. A normal period should not exceed six days (usually three to five), and there should not be more loss than will *soak* three towels a day. There should also be no clots. Menorrhagia is a sign of something wrong in the womb or the body's hormone balance. It may be due to fibroids which sometimes grow in the muscle of the womb (*see* FIBROIDS) or it may be a symptom of womb infection or polyps. It also occurs with some blood disorders, anaemia for instance and in myxoedema (*see* MYXOEDEMA, GOITRE). In some girls the periods are heavy at the time of their commencement at puberty, but the condition usually settles to normal in a few months. If allowed to continue over a number of months excessive blood loss may lead to anaemia, so medical advice should *always* be sought. Most women know what their normal loss should be, and if this increases they should consult their doctor if a month on iron tablets, such as Ferrograd C, does not help.

Menstruation.

A monthly discharge of blood-stained fluid from the womb – known as the period. The womb lining undergoes a continuous cycle of changes. It is gradually built up, and becomes thickened, ready to receive a fertilised ovum but if conception does not take place this lining disintegrates leading to the blood-stained loss. Usually a cycle takes about 28 days, so that the periods should occur at this interval. In some they are painless, but often there is a little pain in the low abdomen and some backache, especially the first day. Sometimes considerable pain is felt, known as dysmenorrhoea (*see* DYSMENORRHOEA) and this calls for medical advice. External sanitary pads can be worn to absorb the flow but many women of all ages prefer the convenience of a tampon designed to fit inside the vagina. They come in different sizes and the smallest will fit easily through the hymen of almost any young girl. They expand snugly in the vaginal space and cannot "get lost" or float about the body.

Some girls start their periods at ten or eleven – others not till sixteen or seventeen. If there is no sign of a period by sixteen, have a word with your doctor. Usually it is just a case of patience but occasionally there are minor disorders that can be put right (e.g. an imperforate hymen).

All indoor and outdoor activities should be carried on as normal during menstruation and it is not an excuse for a rest from gymnastics or hockey.

If conception occurs the membrane does not break up, and therefore the periods stop.

Mental Illness.

One person in seven in the U.K. is expected to suffer some form of mental illness in their lives and hundreds of thousands will attempt suicide, mostly unsuccessfully.

Subnormal intelligence, autism, senility and disorders arising from bodily causes like accidents, tumours, brain damage, etc., are not covered here.

As in physical illness, the disorder can vary from the trivial and tolerable to the distressing and debilitating. In a relatively mild illness where the patient has good insight into his condition, it is known as a *neurosis*. A severe illness in which the patient may have no insight into the absurdity of some of his thoughts (e.g. he has lost touch with reality), is known as a *psychosis*. This requires urgent specialist treatment.

Although an illness may be diagnosed, for example, as depression or anxiety, there may be a mixture of several conditions present. For instance a phobia, which is an irrational fear, may occur by itself or as one feature of a more extensive illness.

Symptoms of mental illness are legion, and include feelings of apathy, depression, anxiety, and obsessions, compulsions, phobias, delusions, undue excitement or verbal or physical aggression (due to fear or guilt) etc. A *phobia* or irrational fear may relate to an open space (agoraphobia), confined spaces (claustrophobia), darkness, certain animals etc. *Obsessed* subjects find their minds compelled unhealthily to circulate on one topic. Patients can deteriorate, and develop *delusions* (see also HALLUCINATION), perhaps believing for example that they will grow a third set of teeth. Where normal fears of inflation, bombs and war, being raped etc. blow up to irrational size, this could be described as an *anxiety state*.

Depression is common, victims seeing no light at the end of the tunnel, and perhaps sitting around in misery. Symptoms can include inability to cope, lack of sense of humour, slow thinking, indecisiveness, lack of normal spontaneous behaviour, sleep disturbance and feelings of unworthiness. *The danger of this is that it can lead to thoughts of suicide*, and so urgent medical attention is needed. The depressed in the U.K. can also ring *The Samaritans* (number in local phone book) who treat everything in complete confidence.

Causes of Mental Illness

Stress or pressure is a common cause. We say "He blew his top", which indicates prolonged breaking of health rules; e.g. too much work, play or perhaps, *both*. Unemployment may cause fear, etc., as does ceaseless worry about insoluble problems and *guilt feelings*. *Conflict* about conscience-squaring behaviour is common as are fears over broken love-lives, and *inferiority feelings*. Sex difficulties can be serious as may be temporary upsets due to menopause or operation.

Hormone imbalance (e.g. Menopause), real or *imagined* physical illnesses, can distort the mind. Money problems, bereavement, frustration, jealousy, loneliness, etc., may harm the mental function. Nightmares, headaches, exhaustion, poor concentration, long silences, self-pity are warning smoke-signals.

Sane or Mad?

With billions of thoughts whirling in our heads, people fall between being normal and abnormal, at times leaning one way then the other with no dividing line. It is a question of degree; often luck, whether one cracks-up or copes. *Every person has a breaking point* – if sufficient strain is applied.

Cures for mental illness

There is misunderstanding and prejudice in this field. Some methods of treatment work for one patient, others for another.

There are many schools of thought on this subject. Some biochemists think that the best results should come eventually from using monitored drugs, as advances are made in understanding the chemistry of the brain. As they see it, troubles arise largely from upsets in your chemistry, accidents etc., so treatment should be mainly physical, any psychotherapy being a bonus.

Most psychiatrists in the U.K. adopt an open-minded approach to treatment, and use a mixture of physical treatments (drugs and Electro Convulsive Therapy – see E.C.T.) and psychotherapy – judging each case on its merits.

The analytical school believes in long-term deep probing into the mind without any physical help. It is costly and impracticable for the severely ill, but may be helpful in neurotic states.

Whatever treatment is decided on, it must be with the agreement of the patient.

The stigma – get rid of it.

Despite proof that *no-one is above the risk of breakdown*, so instinctive is the dread of mental illness that the *stigma* survives, and is *still the biggest hindrance to recovery*.

People connect breakdowns with subnormal intelligence and violence, not appreciating that these are different. Normally in the *stress* breakdowns there is no abnormality and the theory that all such illnesses recur is untrue. A broken leg may be stronger where mended, *so a mind reborn can be better than ever*.

Psychology books which alarm are best avoided by the layman.

A *nervous breakdown* is a lay term and has no precise medical meaning. In fact, it occurs whenever a person feels unable to carry on with his work or family responsibilities because of the severity or intrusion of mental symptoms. It can take almost any form, and by definition will be helped at least partly by the attitudes of family, friends and workmates.

By way of explaining what occurs I quote from "*What Is A Breakdown?*", a great book:

"Mr Smith has been finding his work more of a trial and had been taking longer . . . when he was confronted . . . he went deathly pale, then burst into tears. Afterwards he would not speak to anyone and did not appear to know where he was. He was sent home . . ."

Here is another quotation from what is perhaps the

greatest book* on the subject which, if anything will, should remove the stigma.

Test Your Own Mental Health

"Suffering would be avoided if the notion that no-one is to blame for the occurrence of mental illness could be accepted. Mental illness is not a sign of individual debility. It is not the fault of parents, teachers, siblings, neighbours, lovers or friends . . . all of society is to blame and all of society is blameless."

Treatment with drugs

If you are worried about the length of time you have been taking a certain drug, ask your doctor about this directly. There is probably a good reason such as the expected length of the illness or its liability to recurrence. Keep in touch with your doctor and report improvements as well as deterioration. Don't ignore follow up appointments.

Importance of self-help

This is a neglected field of medicine. The doctor-patient relationship is vital, and it is wise to try to keep the patient carrying on his normal life. The *partly*-cured patient can often recover 100% by self-help, or with help from friends or relatives.

More serious troubles

More serious breakdowns usually need much help but there are instances of spontaneous cure, for faith and time (the greatest healers) often pull off a cure while a psychiatrist is still struggling. Even in after-operation depression there is a psychological basis; at some point due to weakness, etc., the mind says "I cannot bear more" and depres-

---

*WHAT IS A NERVOUS BREAKDOWN? by A.R.K. Mitchell. A booklet published by the British Medical Association, Tavistock Square, London, WC1 (35p).
*TEST YOUR OWN MENTAL HEALTH. 192 pages. A self-evaluation workbook and self-cure programme by Wm. Gladstone, uniform and in the same series with the book, published by ELLIOT RIGHT WAY BOOKS, LOWER KINGSWOOD, TADWORTH, SURREY, KT20 6TD, U.K.

sion starts. Many breakdowns surface quickly, but cures can be rapid too.

We can brain-wash ourselves sick but we can brain-wash ourselves back to health. This is not realised by many doctors.

Feelings of "guilt"

Some disturbed people may act a part to save face, and must not be sneered at. Suppose someone feels guilty of greed, bullying, laziness, etc. He must rectify this by casting out such thoughts if he is sure they are wrong, but, if not, by being unselfish, kind or trying harder.

The acting is an escape and includes pretending to be more ill or believing the cause of the crack-up is physical. The patient need not despise himself or be despised; he is not malingering – the odds got too numerous for him to fight and he needs help. It is easier for his family to explain to others that he is suffering from some named illness causing depression, head pains, etc. This keeps the stigma at bay.

Feeling inferior is common and sufferers must either be content with their position, or change the situation by doing battle. One should achieve one's own ambitions but not be pushed by others. Be yourself and let fools be copycats. Healthy minds accept reality.

Lack of space does not allow details of serious mental illnesses (see Test Your Own Mental Health). It matters little how chronic, long or grave the trouble, if the undernoted conditions are met, permanent recovery should follow.

1. The patient must want to be persuaded to want help.
2. A sufferer must look by himself or with help into the parts of his mind he has tried to forget, dig them out and get rid of any rubbishy thinking. Fear is the basis of the problem; nightmares, loss of concentration, insomnia, inability even to speak, obsession or delusions, etc., are only symptoms. Good doctors recognize this and try to pull out the roots from which the illness grows.
3. Once a patient decides to fight, the darkest clouds can clear, sometimes suddenly, more often with a few relapses.

The mind can put itself out of action by unhealthy

thought. Sufferers must learn to understand the incredible healing power of positive, cheerful thinking and actions, which block out negative ones by taking their place. The seriously ill will need faith in a doctor acceptable to the invalid and probably the co-operation of friends to help him for a few days to keep his mind off his illness.

4. In chronic cases it may have to be explained to the sufferer, perhaps over and over again, possibly for days or weeks *and perhaps tenaciously*, where and how his thinking is unreal and sick. Once these psychological home-truths have sunk in, the patient understands that his illness is *self*-punishment. Then it must be explained that he can return to happy living, and recovery is hastened. He may have to change jobs or live in a new area, or compromise by adjusting his life-style to meet his needs.

In rare instances if a patient is thought to be dangerous to himself or others, call the Police, doctor or social worker as they have legal powers: avoid being left alone with the patient and try to humour him.

Retention of Sanity

Geniuses tend to eat, sleep and drink their subject. Some get away with it, others become obsessed and their lives difficult. Broadly, being a genius is unhealthy. For the majority of people, then, it is wise to try and be conventional, as this makes life easier. The wisdom of being normal is seen when it is realised that mental conditions can be "infectious". Who would have believed almost a thousand people in Guyana would take poison, some forced, others willingly, to please cult leader Jim Jones.

Doing too much can bring trouble. Man is a social animal and should have friends and regular relaxation to preserve sanity. The greater the speed at which a person lives, the more likely he is to drive himself "round the bend". Recreate mind health through recreation or change – even if it is to do a kindness like helping a neighbour.

Among old sayings and expressions which are warnings and well worth pondering are "men make rods for their own backs", "a chip on his shoulder", "flying off the handle" and "mountains out of molehills". The last is one of the most common causes of mental illness. Narrow escapes from madness, often more by luck than by judgement, cover millions of people, so no-one should sneer at others with problems.

To stand back and see ourselves as we *are* is essential for mental health. *If stress strikes*, *get rid of it* by removing the strains one by one until mind balance returns but this must not be taken to excess. As a watch must be balanced to be perfect, so the human brain.

Family rows are a source of conflict, and a person who walks out and "slams the door" is wise because it allows people to "let off steam".

A wife may have been told of her husband's unfaithfulness whilst abroad, and one can imagine her brooding on it and becoming obsessed. Perhaps it was true; more likely the untrue gossip of some jealous woman. In this as in similar situations, remember the old saying that "to err is human, to forgive divine".

Probably the greatest preventative of mental illness is humour. Those who can say perhaps they were treated badly because they deserved to be, or maybe they failed to make friends because they did not bother enough, are obviously pretty healthy. After all, "a little nonsense now and then is relished by the wisest men". (*See* MANIA, PARANOIA, SCHIZOPHRENIA, ANXIETY, E.C.T., DEPRESSION.)

Migraine.

A condition in which the patient suffers recurrent severe headaches. These often run in families, and tend to affect the intelligent. The attacks vary from three or four a year to one a week. In migraine the blood vessels to the brain constrict and then dilate. During constriction at the beginning of an attack, the patient sees flashes, or coloured shapes, and following this is a severe headache, often confined to one half of the head and face. The period of pain corresponds to the period of dilatation of the blood vessels. Tablets such as Effergot which constrict the blood vessels, can if given soon enough, avert the worst of an attack. Vomiting not infrequently occurs at the height of an attack, which usually lasts for from 24 to 48 hours. Suppositories such as Cafergot are useful when vomiting precludes the use of tablets. If the migraine persists the patient is usually best in bed. Two more doses of Effergot may be given at half hour intervals although some find simple analgesics such as Claradin just as helpful. Sometimes elimination of articles such as cheese, chocolate, oranges and red wine from the diet will effect a cure but often it is difficult to pinpoint the offending item. There are tablets which may reduce the incidence of attacks but these need to be taken regularly. Medical advice is needed by frequent sufferers.

Miscarriage. (*See* ABORTION, BIRTH)

Mongolism. (*Down's Syndrome*)

A term used to describe a disorder due to the presence of an extra chromosome in the nuclei of all the body cells. (Chromosomes are coiled threads present in the centre of all body cells and bearing the genes which determine our hereditary characteristics.) The patient has slanting eyes and other physical signs which make the condition easily diagnosed at birth. There is some associated mental retardation but mongols generally are lovable children who can fit well into their family background. After special education they can usually work in sheltered workshops.

The extra chromosome in Down's Syndrome can occur in two ways. With older mothers around forty or so it is thought that the age of the egg is responsible. Young mothers who have mongol babies are generally found on testing to "carry" the extra chromosome attached to the normal one in all their body cells; they suffer no ill effects from this themselves. The young mothers run a risk of having further mongol children although this can be more precisely determined by tests in a genetic counselling clinic. Your family doctor will refer you if necessary.

Mouth Breathing. (*See* ADENOIDS)

Multiple Sclerosis.

A disease of the nervous system in which patches of the protective covering of nerve fibres are worn away piecemeal. The cause is not definitely known. It affects young adults of both sexes and the course is variable. It may start with a temporary defect of vision or pins and needles in one limb. The symptoms tend to improve considerably at first and may be very few and infrequent. Some sufferers have remarkably little disability other than a little clumsiness and weakness after many years. Others follow a more rapidly progressive course and become gradually paraplegic, relying on wheelchairs. Even so periods of improvement can occur. The arm movements tend to be retained. There is no cure yet but some patients are helped by steroids and sunflower seed oil has also seemed beneficial. Physiotherapy helps patients to make the most of their good muscles which must be kept as active as possible.

Newly diagnosed patients can take heart that they may have one of the slow forms of the illness in which serious disabilities may not happen for thirty years or more. Research into causes and treatment continues.

Mumps. (*See* ORCHITIS)

One of the acute infections of childhood, caused by a virus, which affects the salivary glands. These glands produce saliva, and are situated in the neck, one beneath each ear and two under the chin two inches or so from the midline on either side. The glands most often affected are beneath the ears, and pain, particularly on chewing, is often the first symptom. There is usually fever, and after a day or two the glands become swollen. Both sides may be affected together, or often one side first to be followed by the other a day or so later. The incubation period of the infection – the interval between contact and the disease developing – is usually about three weeks but may be four. The swelling lasts one to three weeks, and the patient should be kept apart from others (particularly from young men who may develop testicular inflammation) until the swelling has completely gone. He should be kept in bed until the temperature has settled, and is best given a very soft diet during the early stages since chewing is often painful.

Antiseptic mouthwashes such as Oraldene are soothing. Occasionally other glands are affected, including the sex glands. In males particularly the testes may become swollen, a condition known as *orchitis*, and a watch should be kept for this complication, which will call for a further period of rest in bed. It is for this reason that it is unwise to allow a child to be up and about with mumps while still feverish. In all cases the doctor must be notified.

Murmur. (*See* HEART DISEASE)

Extra sound heard in addition to the normal "lub-dub" of heart beats. In children this is often of no significance so mothers should be reassured if their doctor is satisfied about this. Special tests can be performed if there is any doubt about the cause and the very few found to have heart defects can usually be treated very successfully.

Muscular Dystrophy.

A group of hereditary disorders in which the muscles gradually become weaker due to a defect in metabolism. There are different forms but one common type affects mainly boys in the first five years of life. The condition progresses so that eventually the child is confined to a wheelchair and rarely lives beyond twenty as the breathing muscles are involved. Milder forms of dystrophy occur. Research is going on into the cause and treatments. At present physiotherapy is the mainstay of treatment. Young couples with a family history of muscular dystrophy can have genetic counselling as to the precise risks. Ask your doctor about this. An expectant mother from an "at risk" family can have a test done at the fifteenth week of pregnancy to establish the sex of the baby. If it is a boy there is an even chance of his being affected and she may wish to have termination of pregnancy. A girl will not be affected but can "carry" the disorder. Let us hope more research will come to light on treatment of this distressing condition.

Muscular Rheumatism (*includes fibrositis*).

A vague term used to describe various aches and pains in muscles and soft tissues and due to a variety of causes. Most cases are associated with minor degrees of arthritis or ligament strain in nearby joints – such as the neck, shoulders, hips and knee. The pain is felt in the fleshy muscular area rather than in the deeper ligaments and bones. Others are due to chronic strain as in the lumbar muscles following gardening – lumbago. Rheumatism due to over-use of the muscles needs a short rest, plenty of heat and two soluble aspirins three times a day. Rheumatism due to chronic conditions in joint and ligaments needs as much mobility brought to the area as possible. Rubbing with liniment is helpful. Keep all the joints moving and keep active in general. Soluble aspirin and an appropriate support pad such as a Seton Arthro-pad will allow all the movement to continue with great benefit all round. Supports are not intended for permanent use as they could weaken muscles – wear for a few days while pain is severe. (*See* ARTHRITIS.)

A very important form of rheumatism is *polymyalgia rheumatica*. Symptoms are dramatic and prompt treatment is required as blindness due to arteritis can be a complication if untreated. (*See* ARTERITIS.) An elderly lady finds that her upper arms and thighs become so stiff and painful that she can hardly move and may be literally "stuck" on a chair. There is often no history of previous "rheumatism" or "arthritis". She needs a doctor urgently as blood tests will prove the diagnosis and the need is for steroids. She should be miraculously better in no time and hopefully will avoid the eye complications that cause blindness. Treatment is needed for six months to a year – not less.

Myasthenia Gravis.

The name of an uncommon disease, in which the messages from the brain to various muscles are not properly passed on, so that the muscles affected become weak. The face is often involved, so that the eyelids droop and the patient is unable to laugh or smile. The cause is a fault at the junction between muscle and nerve which becomes blocked to the "chemical messenger", which ought to stimulate it, causing the muscles to move. Treatment consists of giving "excess chemical messenger" (Mestinon) to overcome the block. This often results in a great improvement; in other cases a cure may be brought about by an operation on a gland in the chest called the *thymus* which is not working properly in this disease.

Myocarditis.

Inflammation of the heart muscle. It may complicate several virus diseases, and often accompanies an attack of rheumatic fever. (*See* HEART DISEASE *and* RHEUMATIC FEVER.)

Myxoedema.

A disorder of the thyroid gland where there is insufficient secretion of thyroxine. The body becomes sluggish, there is increase in fat. The hair becomes coarse, the mental processes slow and the skin dry and scaly. It can be cured by Thyroxine tablets. (*See* GOITRE.)

Heavy periods in women and anaemia also occur.

N

Naevus. (*See* BIRTHMARK)

Nails. (*Nail Biting*)

Nails are often affected by the general health, and can indicate anaemia. After a serious illness ridges may appear, which grow out as health returns. Brittle nails may be a symptom of ill health. Nail biting is often a distressing nervous habit in children. Scolding usually has little effect since the habit is mostly instinctive. Punishment upsets the child further so that nail biting becomes more and not less pronounced. The nails should be kept short so that there is little encouragement to bite them. It is best not to make too much of the matter, as the habit is nearly always one which the child grows out of, especially if success is rewarded.

Nephritis.

The medical term for inflammation of the kidneys. It may occur as an acute condition (*see* ACUTE) when recovery is often complete, but sometimes the disease becomes chronic and lowers the general health considerably. The reader should consult the article on KIDNEY DISEASES.

Nettlerash. (*Urticaria*)

One of the allergic diseases (*see* ALLERGY, HAY FEVER). It is due to irritation of the skin by some foreign substance – often in the diet. Red weals develop on the skin which irritate, and have white tops. One common cause of urticaria is eating shellfish, and sometimes, especially in children, eggs may cause the condition. The rash does not usually last long, and the best treatment is to avoid the substance which causes the attack. Calamine lotion is soothing, and antihistamine tablets, such as Piriton cure rapidly. (Warning to drivers – antihistamines cause drowsiness, so avoid driving while taking them.)

Neuralgia. (*See* NEURITIS)

Neuritis.
Inflammation of a nerve, which is not common. It may occur when a nerve passes through inflamed tissue and certain metallic poisons such as lead, which may contaminate drinking water, are capable of setting up a neuritis. It can also be due to virus infection and in multiple sclerosis (*see* MULTIPLE SCLEROSIS) many widespread areas of neuritis occur. There are two sorts of nerves – those which carry sensations (pain, etc.) back to the brain, and those which carry messages to move the muscles. In neuritis, both functions may be disturbed, so that the muscles in the affected part become weak, and sensations disturbed, resulting in pain, numbness or sometimes "pins and needles". The condition is often confused with *neuralgia* which is the occurrence of pain in the area served by a particular nerve. The condition is often due to an "over-flow", so to speak, from a small painful focus. Thus a diseased tooth may set up a neuralgia of the whole face. The pain from neuralgia can often be lessened by aspirin, but it is always wisest to see a doctor for face or temple pain as often there is some underlying cause to be put right before the trouble will settle completely. Neuritis is sometimes confused with ARTERITIS.

Night Blindness.
The sensitive part at the back of the eye (the retina) has two components – one for day vision, including colours; the other for vision at night, where there is no appreciation of colour; only of shade and shape. The efficient working of the latter depends upon a good supply of Vitamin A (*see*

PAGE 9). If this is lacking in the diet, night blindness may result.

Night Sweats.

Excessive sweating at night is often a sign of a raised temperature and can be caused by a variety of conditions. Infections such as tooth abscess and sinusitis are probably the commonest. Night sweats also occur in thyrotoxicosis (*See* GOITRE) and in anxiety states. Although much rarer nowadays TUBERCULOSIS is an important cause. *Recurrent* night sweats should be reported to your doctor for investigation.

Nit. (*See* LICE)

Nose Bleeding. (*See* HAEMORRHAGE)

N.S.U. *(non-specific urethritis, non-specific genital infection)*.

Any inflammation of the urethra (outlet from the bladder) in which have been excluded such diseases as GONORRHOEA, SYPHILIS and infection (*See* VAGINITIS) by larger germs such as trichomonas and monilia (THRUSH).

It is now the commonest venereal disease in the U.K. Symptoms may include pain on passing water, soreness of the parts and discharge, but are milder than in gonorrhoea and the symptoms are usually completely absent in the female. About 50% of NSU cases are thought to be caused by a virus-like germ called chlamydia. Unfortunately chlamydia can cause serious infection in the eyes of newborn babies, as can gonorrhoea.

Treatment is not perfect but consists of tetracycline antibiotics for four to six weeks. This is different from the usual treatments for *cystitis* (a different illness) so any patient who suspects that pain on passing water may be due to sexual contact should always mention this to his or her doctor or attend a special clinic. In spite of treatment a few men develop serious complications such as arthritis and inflammation of the eyes and it is not absolutely certain that treatment of female contacts will prevent development of eye inflammation in new-born babies.

The only definite way to avoid these ills is not to have casual sex where you cannot be sure that your partner is free of infection.

Nystagmus.

The name of a condition in which there is a rapid to and fro movement of the eyeballs. It can be seen in normal persons who have spun round until giddy and it usually passes off in less than a minute. Sometimes, in disease of the brain, or in people who have worked long in a poor light, like miners, the control of the eye movements becomes disturbed so that nystagmus occurs all the time. In modern well-lit mines this should no longer occur. Some families have a tendency to this condition for no obvious reason and their sight is not impaired. Your doctor will advise you if any abnormal eye movements you may have noted are of any serious significance.

O

Obesity.

Excessive weight is unsightly and detrimental to the health as it imposes unnecessary strain on the body. In a few cases, the condition may be due to a glandular disorder; and the increase in weight which often accompanies the "change of life" in women is due in part to the same cause (*See* MENOPAUSE).

Usually, however, the cause boils down to mathematics. Too much fat-producing food, too little exercise to burn it up, so the fat accumulates. Unfortunately some people burn up their food at a slower rate than others and do have to eat a much more restricted diet to achieve a reasonable weight. In spite of treatments which are advertised, there is no safe, easy road to weight reduction. The key is to restrict fat-producing foods so that no more fat is stored, and what has become stored is burnt up. The chief offenders are the sugary and starchy foods which become converted to fat if not used. Sugar, sweets, bread, potatoes, jams and pastry must be reduced to a minimum by anyone wishing to lose weight. Fish, green vegetables and fruit may be eaten *ad lib*. Meat should not exceed 6oz of lean daily and butter, margarine and milk should be restricted. Cheese and eggs may be substituted for meat and fish.

A straightforward régime without fads may be summarised as follows. Give up all sugar, jams, sweets and pastry and do not use more milk than is required in the tea. Cut potatoes to one medium sized a day not cooked with fat. Have one slice of wholemeal bread or two biscuits such as "Ryvita" instead. Eat plenty of fish and a daily total of 8oz of protein foods such as cheese, lean meat and lean bacon. Fill up on green vegetables, particularly salads in season, and fruits. Do not be tempted to "nibble" between meals. The more daily exercise taken, within reason, the better, as this helps to burn the fat already accumulated. Obesity is a long-term problem which requires a long-term solution. Two or three weeks "dieting" is useless. A complete and permanent change in dietary and exercise habits is needed. Do not ask your doctor for "slimming" tablets. The only ones available cut down your appetite; they do not "slim" you and their effect tends to wear off.

Contrary to popular belief excess fluid is not a cause of overweight. Except in serious disease even the most bloated of us is only carrying about seven pounds too much fluid but probably about three stone too much fat. Most of the excess fluid will disappear along with the fat if you stick to the above diet, as long as salt intake is kept to a minimum (a little in cooking only). It is no good "starving" as the bowel needs volume to help the "fat stuff" to pass. Eat lots of fruits and vegetables to provide the fibre needed to keep the bowels right.

Obstruction.

Term commonly used in relation to the bowel when blockage by, for instance, tumour, or adhesions from a previous operation, causes intense pain due to the increased efforts of the bowel muscle to expel the cause of the block. There is usually constipation and later on vomiting develops as the intestinal contents build up behind the source of the obstruction. Treatment is usually by emergency operation to remove the obstructions. The combination of severe abdominal pain, constipation and vomiting requires urgent medical help.

In elderly people extreme constipation can lead to this condition and treatment is by bowel washout. This is rare in other age groups.

Oedema.

Collection of fluid within the body tissues. (Sometimes archaicly called dropsy.) Due to gravity, the lower parts of the body are those most affected, so that ankles, then legs, and later the abdomen become distended. Swollen legs will show a little pit when pressed with the finger. There are various causes. It may be associated with HEART DISEASE when circulation becomes so sluggish that fluid leaks from the blood vessels into the tissues. It can be due to KIDNEY DISEASE, when the kidneys are unable to eliminate excess water which accumulates. Some degree of swelling of the ankles especially after middle age is common and does not necessarily indicate serious illness. Overweight is a common and remediable cause. In pregnancy some women develop swollen ankles. Treatment of oedema includes rest, restriction of salt (which "holds onto" the fluid) and the use of tablets or injections to eliminate water (diuretics). Where oedema is due to heart disease digoxin may also be needed.

Old Age.

If one lives long enough mind and body deteriorate but probably the way to prolong happy living is as far as possible never think of your age *in years* at all.

It may be that those who are optimistic and do not adopt the attitude that they have to give up things, or stay in, because it is "too wet or cold" remain healthiest. *Keep exercising mind and body* and develop interests to compensate for those which have to be given up. If you cannot play tennis at 60 consider bowls, rambling, etc. Never think: "I must not buy a coat as I may not need it". *That,* is the philosophy of death. Every age has its compensations and many people in their 90s still enjoy life. With modern medicines there is much that can be done to delay the effects of age and reduce the risk that you may have to enter hospital. The ability to adjust *physically and mentally* is probably the most likely way to hit a century. To all who say "I do not want to live that long," a good reply is, "if you do, you will".

Operations. (*See* ANAESTHESIA)

Orchitis.

Inflammation of the testes, the male sex glands. It usually results from an attack by germs and may occur as a complication of mumps. Another cause is a venereal infection, especially gonorrhoea. The symptoms are pain and swelling in the testes, and if these occur there should be no time lost in seeing a doctor. In a young boy swelling and pain can be due to twisting of the testicle (*See* TORSION OF TESTICLE) and urgent operation is required to save the testis. Men who suffer orchitis – a rather frightening illness, should not be too afraid. The enormous swelling of the testis can be helped by various drugs and normally the gland returns to its usual function without any loss of virility or fertility.

Osteoarthritis.

The "wear and tear" type of arthritis in which the joint surfaces become roughened, irregular and painful. It may be aggravated by excess weight or previous injury and is common in the weight-bearing joints such as hip and knee. For treatment see ARTHRITIS.

Osteomyelitis. (*Bone Infection*)

Infection within the bone cavity. Germs from some focus of infection which may not be obvious may, particularly after injury, gain entry to the blood stream and thence to the interior of a bone. The condition most commonly occurs in the knee – towards the ends of the bones above or below the joint, but can occur in any other bones. The infection trapped within the bones, causes excruciating pain, and a high temperature. Attempts to move the affected part increases the pain and the child (for children are usually affected) will remain unusually still. Antibiotics may cure but sometimes it is necessary to operate to release the pus. Occasionally the tubercle bacillus is the cause and it is then known as tuberculous osteomyelitis. Treatment in this case requires anti-tuberculous drugs which are very effective. Antibiotics have largely prevented the long-term effects which included destruction of large areas of bone and recurrences of discharge from sinuses in the limbs but the condition still needs urgent treatment in the early stages.

Otitis Externa.

Inflammation of the outer ear canal leading down to the eardrum. It causes itching, pain and discharge. Treatment is by eardrops which soothe and contain antibiotic or anti-fungus agents. You will need medical advice.

Otitis Media.

Inflammation of the middle ear usually due to infection which has spread from the nose or throat. EARACHE, especially in children, is frequently due to otitis media and early medical attention is needed so that antibiotics can be prescribed if necessary. In this way complications like MASTOIDITIS, chronic discharge and DEAFNESS may be avoided.

Otorrhoea.

Discharge from the ear. It can occur in OTITIS EXTERNA and also in OTITIS MEDIA if the eardrum bursts due to pressure from pus building up in the middle ear. This type of drum perforation usually heals quickly, but in neglected cases the perforation may be permanent and the discharge recur from time to time. (See DEAFNESS.)

Ovaries.

The female sex glands, which lie inside the abdominal cavity, one on each side above the womb. They produce the ova, or eggs, which after uniting with a sperm, are capable of growing into a baby. One ovum is usually produced approximately every 28 days, about midway between the times of the periods, and the lining of the womb is increased in thickness to receive it. (See GLANDS, HORMONES, INFERTILITY, MENOPAUSE, MENSTRUATION.)

Ovarian Cyst.

A fluid-filled swelling which can develop in one or both ovaries. There may be no symptoms unless it becomes twisted to cause pain. Cysts may sometimes cause irregular periods and the "chocolate" cysts of ENDOMETRIOSIS are associated with painful periods. Sometimes cysts are only noticed when they become large enough to cause an increase in girth. An ovarian cyst requires medical investigation as occasionally it may contain a tumour. (*See* DYSMENORRHOEA.)

P

Pacemaker. (*See* HEART DISEASE)

Pain.

A warning signal. The body is supplied with a network of nerves which carry messages to the brain, and when these are irritated or injured we feel pain. Pain lets us know something is wrong, and serves to protect the injured or diseased part from further damage since a painful part is usually moved as little as possible. In injury the body may not wait for the brain to analyse the message before taking action. We have all had the experience of touching something hot and feeling the sudden jerk as the hand jumps away almost before the pain is felt. This is brought about by the spinal cord where the pain signals are "short-circuited" as it were and made to move the muscles *before* they reach the brain. This is known as a *reflex*, and may occur even when a person is unconscious. Blinking when something approaches the eye is example of a reflex. Whatever its nature pain is an indication of something amiss. It may be only trivial, and we all suffer from aches and pains which do not last long. Any severe pain, or any which is persistent should not be ignored. See your doctor and get him to treat you.

Pallor.

Pronounced paleness or pallor may simply be a matter of complexion or may indicate a shortage of the red colouring matter (haemoglobin) in the blood. The latter is more likely if the lips and red membrane inside the eyelids are also pale. (*See* ANAEMIA.)

Palpitations.

Normally the heart beats steadily and we are unaware of its action. Sometimes when the beating becomes quicker or irregular we are aware of a fluttering sensation in the chest known as palpitations. It occasionally occurs in heart disease and thyrotoxicosis (*See* GOITRE) when the heart is working less well than normal, but usually palpitations are not due to any serious disorder. They often accompany an emotional upset, and can be brought on by excess cigarette smoking. Lay people are often unduly worried by palpitations and feel something serious has gone wrong. If the symptom persists for any time medical advice should certainly be sought, but in most cases there is no cause for anxiety. Worry and stress make us unduly aware of the *normal* action of the heart as well as tending to speed it up. This is the commonest cause of palpitations. If the doctor tells you all is well, do not worry about the condition. (*See* PULSE.)

Pancreas.

An organ lying behind the stomach. It produces digestive juices which pass along a duct into the duodenum. Small areas of its surface (islets) produce insulin which is poured directly into the blood stream to control the level of blood sugar.

Paralysis.

The loss of voluntary movement of a part of the body – a loss of the power to move the muscles concerned. It may be associated with a loss or disorder of sensation, but this is not necessarily the case since the two sets of nerves, motor and sensory, are separate (*See* NEURITIS). Paralysis may be a symptom of disease or injury to that part of the brain, which controls movements (e.g. a STROKE), to the spinal cord which passes on the messages, or to the nerves themselves (e.g. NEURITIS). (One of the commonest causes of spinal paralysis nowadays is injury due to motor car accident.) Unfortunately, most types of paralysis (except where due to fear, when it is fleeting) which have persisted for any length of time do not usually recover completely, because injured nerve cells cannot be replaced. However, there is often some remaining function in the part concerned, and by special exercises designed to make use of this the patient can often do much to overcome the disability.

Paranoia.

A type of mental sickness, characterised by suspicion of being victimised. It may develop quickly or slowly and may persist or remit. One cause of the illness could be loneliness. The patient tends to brood a lot. Mild cases may merely be considered eccentric or bad tempered people. By the time a doctor is seen, a sufferer may, in rare cases, be deluded enough to believe that God has chosen him to do something, possibly something terrible. It can be difficult but *essential* to get the patient to see a doctor. So tenacious can the patient's views be that some of those close to him may imagine them correct. Specialist treatment is often required.

In the early stages, various modern drug treatments of one kind or another are very often useful, and may need to be continued for some time. Psychotherapy may be of use later on. The outlook should be excellent if a doctor can be found of an acceptable wavelength to the patient. A new job or improved life conditions may be advisable. (*See* E.C.T., MANIA, MENTAL ILLNESS *and* SCHIZOPHRENIA.)

Parasite.

A plant or animal which lives upon or within another living organism causing damage and giving no benefit. Examples of parasitic diseases are malaria (*See* MALARIA) in which the parasite is transferred from mosquito to man, and amoebic dysentery (*See* DYSENTERY) in which the parasite is acquired from contaminated food or water.

Parathyroids.

Four small glands arranged in two pairs near the outer lobes of the thyroid gland in the neck. They produce a hormone which controls calcium metabolism and thus the condition of bones. Too much hormone, e.g. with a tumour of the gland, eventually produces kidney and bone damage. Too little hormone causes defects in teeth, nails, skin and hair and can also cause an acute form of muscular cramp plus pins and needles, known as tetany.

Parkinson's Disease. *(Paralysis Agitans, shaking palsy)*

A condition in which the muscles become stiff and jerky in their action. It is due to disturbance of that part of the brain which controls the smooth working of muscles caused in some cases by hardening of the cerebral arteries. Sufferers are greatly handicapped by the stiffness and tremor, but can often be helped by medicines which help to lessen these symptoms. A breakthrough in treatment was the development of the drug "Levo-dopa" which has been of great value to many. Rarely found in the under-fifties.

Parturition. *(Medical term for child-birth).* (*See* BIRTH)

Penicillin.

This very important drug was discovered by Sir Alexander Fleming – a Scot – at St. Mary's Hospital, London when a mould got into a dish in which bacteria were growing. It was noted at the time that the bacteria were killed by this mould but it was some years before the active ingredient – penicillin – was extracted in sufficient quantity to become the first of the antibiotics (*See* ANTIBIOTICS). Unlike many powerful drugs penicillin is harmless to normal body tissues except in a few patients who are, or become, allergic to it. Mild allergy usually consists of a skin rash, and anyone who has had this should avoid future doses of penicillin at all costs (there are now alternative antibiotics). Penicillin and its modern derivatives ampicillin, flucloxacillin, etc., are still the best treatments for many infections including boils, pneumonia, meningitis, syphilis and gonorrhoea.

Penis.

The male sex organ, containing a canal, the *urethra,* through which urine from the bladder is passed. If this becomes inflamed, as for instance in GONORRHOEA, the condition is known as urethritis. Normally the penis is relaxed, but it contains a special tissue in which are large blood spaces. Under the influence of sexual excitement or sometimes friction these become distended with blood which causes the organ to erect and become stiff. At the end of the sexual act, semen, a fluid containing the male sperms (seed), is discharged via the urethra. Rarely, sexual union is made difficult by a deformity of the penis. The opening at the end of the urethra may lie on the under-surface of the penis (hypospadias) or sometimes the organ is bent over. Successful surgical refashioning or re-shaping is now usually performed in the early years of life and can cure or help in many instances. (*See* BALANITIS, CIRCUMCISION, FORESKIN *and* PHIMOSIS.)

Pericarditis.

The heart is surrounded by a membrane known as the pericardium. Under some circumstances this may become inflamed. There are many causes and the commonest is a range of virus infections. The inflamed membrane may pour out fluid which then collects around the heart, a condition known as *pericardial effusion*. Whatever the cause the condition is serious, and the patient will usually require a long period of rest to allow the infection to subside.

Period. (*See* AMENORRHOEA, BIRTH, MENSTRUATION)

Peritonitis.

Inflammation of the membrane (peritoneum) which lines the abdominal cavity. It is a very serious condition and usually occurs when an infected organ bursts as in APPENDICITIS. Treatment depends on the cause but often includes emergency operation as well as antibiotics. Prevention means treatment of the original trouble (e.g. appendicitis) before this stage is reached. We all get odd tummy aches from time to time but in general any abdominal pain which persists for four hours, especially if there is associated fever and vomiting, needs a doctor's attention. The pain of peritonitis is so severe that it usually causes collapse and, if a doctor cannot be immediately located, dial 999 for an emergency ambulance (in U.K.).

Pernicious Anaemia.

Study the article on ANAEMIA in general. Whereas many anaemias are due to lack of iron, pernicious anaemia is due to lack of vitamin B_{12}, also essential for the manufacture of red blood cells. It is caused by poor absorption from the stomach rather than inadequate diet and occurs in older people where the stomach lining has become thin and unable to deal with this vitamin.

Lack of vitamin B_{12} (cyanocobalamin) also causes damage to nerve cells so that as well as symptoms of anaemia (tiredness, shortness of breath, etc.) the patient may have disturbances of sensation (pins and needles, numbness, etc.) and weakness of the arms and legs. As the patient is unable to absorb vitamin B_{12} from the stomach, treatment is by regular injection. When the condition is first diagnosed injections may be given several times a week. However, after the first week or two they can be reduced to once monthly.

A similar condition arises if the diet is deficient in vitamin B_{12} (rare in the West) or after surgery for peptic ulcer when a part of the stomach is removed. Increased intake of liver is indicated for the former and regular injections of B_{12} for the latter.

Pessary.

Any device placed in the vagina for the purposes of treatment. It may be to support the uterus as in prolapse (*See* PROLAPSE) or to act as a contraceptive (diaphragm pessary) or to treat infection when it can consist of a drug incorporated in a suitably shaped soluble tablet.

Pharyngitis.

Inflammation of the throat often accompanying TONSILLITIS or (if the tonsils have been removed) occurring alone. It may be caused by the streptococcus – the "tonsillitis germ" – or by numerous viruses. Only "strep" throats respond to penicillin. The vast majority of virus-inflamed throats settle in their own good time (about a week) and can be soothed by gargle of glycerine of thymol and soluble aspirin.

Phimosis. (*See* BALANITIS *and* CIRCUMCISION.)

A constriction of the male foreskin. Normally after the age of three it can be pulled back to expose the tip of the penis for purposes of hygiene but sometimes the opening of the foreskin is too narrow. Mothers should not attempt to retract the foreskin before the child is four as scarring can occur in the delicate tissues. Slight adherence of the foreskin in a young boy can often be treated medically by gentle stretching. Where there is genuine phimosis it is usually best to deal with this condition by circumcision, since debris is likely to accumulate beneath the foreskin, resulting in inflammation (BALANITIS). Sometimes a tight foreskin becomes constricted around the head of the penis after it has been pulled back – a condition known as *paraphimosis*. For this, too, circumcision is often the best treatment.

Phlebitis.

Inflammation of a vein. Veins may become inflamed as the result of disease or injury, and the most common situation is in the leg where the cause is often a varicosity of the veins (*See* VARICOSE VEINS). The vein affected becomes hard, and can be felt like a cord beneath the skin. It is often tender and the overlying skin may be inflamed. Consult a doctor, for phlebitis in a superficial vein is liable to spread if not properly treated. He will probably prescribe a supporting bandage, tablets to reduce inflammation and plenty of walking exercise to keep the circulation flowing through the deeper veins of the leg. Outlook usually excellent.

Photophobia.

A term applied when the eyes are unduly sensitive to light. It commonly occurs where the eyes are inflamed, and may be a feature of generalised infections in which the eyes are involved, e.g. MEASLES. It often accompanies any severe headache, and frequently occurs during an attack of MIGRAINE. A serious but less common cause is MENINGITIS when it accompanies headache and neck stiffness. The treatment depends on the cause, but whatever that is, it is always best to avoid bright light and straining the eyes when they are sensitive.

Piles. (*See* HAEMORRHOIDS)

Pink Eye.

The popular name for a bacterial CONJUNCTIVITIS. (*See* EYE, EYESIGHT.)

Pins and Needles. *(Paraethesiae)*

Sensations such as burning and prickling – often in the limbs. It may be due to pressure on the nerve (your arm may "go to sleep" if you lie on it) or it may be due to inflammation as in neuritis (*See* NEURITIS). Often the pricking goes if one alters one's sleeping position to, for example, having an arm behind the back. If these sensations persist see your doctor.

Pleurisy.

Each lung is enclosed in a double layer of thin membrane known as the pleura *(see* FIG. 9, *page 116)*. When it becomes inflamed the condition is known as pleurisy. It is nearly always due to an invasion by germs which may reach the pleura through the bloodstream or from the lung beneath. Thus pleurisy is apt to follow infections of the lung – particularly pneumonia. When the pleura becomes inflamed it often pours out fluid which collects between the two layers, and this is known as a *pleural effusion*. During the early stages, pleurisy is usually accompanied by a sharp pain in the chest on breathing, since the inflamed layers of membrane rub against each other every time a breath is taken. In the later stages, if fluid forms, the pain passes off since the fluid prevents the two layers from coming into contact. However, the presence of the fluid reduces the movement of the lung so that there is often shortness of breath.

Nowadays pleurisy is often due to a number of viruses and there may be little or no associated pneumonia. Treatment is by rest and tablets to reduce pain thus aiding deep breathing. Where pleurisy is due to bacteria it responds well to antibiotics.

Pleurodynia.

A common virus infection (also called *Bornholm disease*) affecting the muscles between the ribs and sometimes causing true pleurisy and pericarditis. Fever and a sharp chest pain on breathing in are the main symptoms. (*See* PLEURISY.)

Pneumoconiosis.

Disease of the lungs in which inhalation of dust causes thickening and scarring in the delicate lung tissues. It used to be an occupational hazard in mining before the introduction of safety measures such as air filters. The end result is persistent shortness of breath and liability to chest infections and other lung disease. Similar reactions occur with exposure to silicon (silicosis) – a hazard among knife grinders – and to *blue* asbestos now banned by most companies (asbestosis).

Pneumonia.

A serious infection of part of the lung causing the normally "spongy" tissue to become solid. There are several varieties of pneumonia depending upon the germ and the parts of the lung affected. Thus *lobar pneumonia* is due to the pneumococcus, which attacks a whole lobe of the lung at once. In BRONCHO-PNEUMONIA, which may be caused by different germs, the infection is more scattered and occurs in patches surrounding the breathing tubes. It follows some other respiratory infection, such as a cold or 'flu, when the patient, instead of recovering, grows worse. There is a pain in the chest if the pleura is involved (*See* PLEURISY), usually a high temperature of 103°F (39½°C) and a cough productive of rusty-looking phlegm. As more of the lung becomes involved, some shortness of breath becomes apparent. There may be a tinge of blueness in face and lips.

Most forms of pneumonia respond rapidly to antibiotic treatment. Pneumonia caused by viruses however does not respond to such treatment and can be dangerous, requiring intensive hospital care, including oxygen.

Pneumothorax.

The term for the presence of air between the layers of the pleura (*See* PLEURISY). Sometimes, when there is disease present and sometimes for no obvious reason a small hole may form in a terminal air passage and allow air to escape, and press on the lung causing it to collapse. In many instances rest alone will allow a lung to expand naturally curing the condition. Occasionally a "tension" pneumothorax develops as air continues to build up in the chest cavity pressing ever harder on the collapsed lung. Emergency treatment in hospital is needed to release the air through a tube inserted through the chest wall. Thereafter treatment is rest as for ordinary pneumothorax.

Poisoning.

Many substances in daily use are harmful and may be taken accidentally, or sometimes deliberately in intended suicide. The most common symptoms are pain in mouth, throat and stomach, vomiting and collapse and undue drowsiness. Later, there is often diarrhoea. A sudden illness in a person previously well should arouse suspicion, and if the victim is questioned it may be found that something out of the ordinary has been taken. The remedy for a poison depends on its nature, but the *general* treatment is usually the same. Call the doctor and let him know that an overdose of medicine or poisoning is suspected. The treatment is very complicated and usually needs expert medical care in hospital. Many first aid procedures can be dangerous. Attempts to make a drowsy or semi-conscious patient vomit should await the arrival of a doctor since *inhalation of vomit into the lungs can easily happen*. Never give a solution of salt. If someone has taken an overdose of tablets keep the bottle to enable the doctor to identify which drug and how much has been taken. Vomited material should also be kept for inspection.

Do not give other medicines or alcohol except to the fully conscious and co-operative patients as below. Drowsiness and coma should be treated by placing the patient in the three quarters prone (i.e. lying on his side) position, making sure the tongue is pulled forwards to maintain a clear airway. Dentures should be removed. Be ready to use artificial respiration (*See* ARTIFICIAL RESPIRATION) if necessary.

(a) *Acids*. These include sulphuric acid (oil of vitriol), hydrochloric acid (spirits of salt), battery acid, nitric acid, soldering fluid, formic acid (kettle descaler) and phenol (carbolic acid). Give a glass of milk mixed with two teaspoons of bicarbonate of soda or the stomach mixture "Asilone", four teaspoons to the fully conscious patient. Do not induce vomiting.

(b) *Alkalis*. The most common are caustics, such as caustic potash, caustic soda and ammonia. A glass of milk mixed, if possible, with beaten white of egg may be given to the conscious patient. Do not induce vomiting.

(c) *Arsenic*. This is present in sheep dip and less commonly nowadays in weedkiller. Vomiting may be induced in the conscious patient by giving two teaspoons of mustard in a glass of water. This should be followed by a glass of milk mixed with two teaspoons of vegetable oil.

(d) *Carbon tetrachloride* (dry cleaning fluid). Give nothing by mouth.

(e) *Paraquat*. This is the most dangerous of the modern weedkillers. Urgent specialist care is vital and the patient should be rushed to the nearest hospital either by emergency ambulance or home transport if quicker. Vomiting may be induced, as for Arsenic (above).

(f) *Overdose of sleeping tablets, tranquillisers or antidepressant drugs*. If the patient is fully conscious, as may be the case within minutes of taking the overdose, induction of vomiting may be tried by two teaspoons of mustard in water. Keep the patient warm whilst awaiting medical aid and be prepared to administer artificial respiration (*See* ARTIFICIAL RESPIRATION) if necessary.

To avoid accidental poisoning, all medicines and other poisonous substances should be kept out of reach of children since they will readily eat tablets experimentally or mistake them for sweets. They will also drink any liquid especially foolishly transferred to a "soft drink" bottle. This is the usual reason for the accidental drinking of household cleaners, carbolic acid and paraquat. A little common sense would prevent these tragedies. Warn children not to eat any berries as it is impossible for them to distinguish the safe from the poisonous.

Poliomyelitis. (*Infantile Paralysis*)

This disease is now fortunately rare in the U.K. and is becoming rarer throughout the world. It is infectious and caused by a virus which gains entry to the intestines via the mouth and stomach. First it produces a vague 'flu-like illness with fever, diarrhoea, headache and limb pains. After two to three days paralysis may develop in some people. As the virus reaches the spinal nerve cells controlling movement this paralysis may affect a single limb or may be extensive and affect the breathing muscles, causing death or the need for mechanically assisted respiration. Avoid exercise in the early stage of the illness as it seems to increase the extent of the subsequent paralysis so rest is vital if there is any suspicion of polio.

Fortunately the development of safe and effective oral vaccines has almost eliminated this disease from Western countries. However, in some tropical and sub-tropical countries it still occurs in small epidemics. Travellers to such countries, including the Mediterranean coast, are advised to be vaccinated or to have booster doses. There is at present a campaign starting to eliminate polio by a world vaccination programme.

Polycythaemia.
Medical term for an uncommon condition where the red cells in the blood are increased above normal. It often causes a ruddy complexion, and may be associated with headaches, and sometimes raised blood pressure. There are medicines which can be taken by mouth to reduce the number of cells to a more normal level.

Polypus.
A small, pear-shaped growth forming on the internal surfaces of the body. Polypi are usually caused by chronic infection and are commonly found in ears or nose. They also occur in women, sometimes, at the *cervix,* the exit from the womb. Polypi are not dangerous in themselves, but may cause irritation and bleed from time to time. They are usually easily removed by a small operation.

Pregnancy.
Pregnancy occurs when the female ovum is fertilised by the sperm and embeds satisfactorily in the lining of the womb. The first indication is usually a stopping of the monthly period though there are other causes (*See* AMENOR-

RHOEA). Any blood loss after pregnancy is confirmed requires medical advice. During the early months there is sometimes a feeling of sickness or vomiting in the morning. The breasts enlarge somewhat and during a first pregnancy the nipples and surrounding skin become darker. After about the third month the abdomen becomes noticeably and progressively larger. The normal duration of pregnancy is nine months, or to be more precise, 40 weeks. The expected date of birth can be calculated thus. Take the first day of the last monthly period, count back three months and add seven days. Thus if the last period started on August 14th the birth would be due on May 21st. Every woman should put herself under the care of her doctor during pregnancy. It is important to have a regular check to see that all is going well, and she will require advice about diet and exercise so that she can remain in good health during pregnancy. The blood pressure needs to be taken regularly to exclude rises which might be harmful. If the blood pressure does rise and if albumen appears in the urine the mother needs complete rest, sometimes in hospital. Occasionally the birth needs to be induced early if rest does not suffice. Cigarette smoking should be given up as it damages the unborn child and is one cause of underweight babies. No medicines other than those deemed necessary and safe by your doctor, should be taken, especially in the first three months, as they can lead to deformities of the baby. Extra iron and vitamins are advisable during pregnancy and can be prescribed by your doctor. If all is going well there is no reason why you cannot continue your job at least until the seven month stage. (*See* BIRTH, BREAST *and* INFANT FEEDING.)

Premature Birth.
A birth before the 37th week and after the 28th week of pregnancy. (*See* ABORTION *and* MISCARRIAGE.)

Premenstrual Tension.
In the ten days or so before a menstrual period many women feel bloated, tense and irritable. In a few this may interfere with their concentration at work, their driving ability and their family life. Studies have shown that badly

affected women have a relative lack of the hormone progesterone, and they may feel much better on progestergen or progesterone treatment. Tablets to eliminate excess fluid help to a lesser extent. It is easy to become too introspective about your menstrual cycle but if there seems to be a definite time relationship between the premenstrual week and *serious* symptoms your doctor may be able to help.

Prolapse.

The falling down or sinking of a part. It can occur with many organs including the back passage but is commonly used to describe "sinking" of the womb into the vagina or bulging of the front and back walls of the vagina. The ligaments supporting the uterus and the tissues of the vagina may be inherently weak in some women and all are stretched during delivery of a baby. There are often no immediate symptoms in the young healthy mother but later, especially around the menopause when the tissues become less resilient, the symptoms of prolapse may appear. Symptoms include a feeling of "something coming down" in the vaginal region. A swelling may be seen or there may be backache and vague lower abdominal discomfort. Difficulty in passing water, accidentally passing water while coughing or sneezing or recurrent cystitis (*See* CYSTITIS) may indicate that the front vaginal wall next to the bladder has dropped. Increasing constipation associated with a vaginal lump may mean that the back vaginal wall is bulging.

Careful attention to post natal exercises in the six weeks after childbirth may prevent the appearance of prolapse years later. These consist simply of tightening up the muscles which stop you passing water when you want to do so. This exercise can be performed twenty times a day as you are doing other jobs including washing up! The reward for doing the exercise may be also increased sex enjoyment. The same exercises may help to control mild prolapse when it first appears. Electrical treatment may also assist by stimulating the muscles. A ring pessary (*See* PESSARY) will control many cases of prolapse but needs regular changing (three to six monthly) by a doctor or nurse and younger women would probably not wish to wear a pessary permanently. Operation to tighten up the ligaments and vaginal wall is probably best for most women. This is done from below so that there is no visible scar. After six to twelve weeks sex relations can be resumed and may even be improved by the tightening up of slack vaginal walls. Extra lubrication (e.g. KY jelly) may be needed at first and perhaps gentle dilatation by the woman's own fingers increasing gradually from one to three. Your gynaecologist will advise on the use of polythene dilators if this proves necessary but often simpler measures suffice.

If fibroids or some other condition is found to co-exist with a prolapse the repair may be combined with a hysterectomy (*See* HYSTERECTOMY) also performed from below.

Prostate.

A gland situated at the outlet of the bladder in men. Disease of the prostate interferes with the flow of urine.

Prostatitis

Inflammation of the gland can occur when germs enter from the urine. This condition causes fever, backache and trouble in passing water. It can also be a cause of general ill-health. Treatment is usually with antibiotics.

Prostate Cancer

A common but easily treated form of cancer which causes difficulty in passing water. The tumour can spread from the prostate into the bones. Treatment is by surgery and by the use of special hormone tablets or injections.

Benign Prostatic Hypertrophy

This is the commonest form of prostate trouble, a simple enlargement of the gland with increasing age.

If your water works are not functioning normally, or if you have pain passing water or discomfort in your bladder or sex organs, it may be something which will pass, but it could be an indication of an enlarged prostate.

If this happens act quickly, do not be shy; it is a common illness, especially in older men. Slight difficulty with the stream can progress to complete inability to empty the bladder, which would need insertion of a catheter (tube). Consult a doctor *immediately,* because delay can cause *serious damage* and/or necessitate a major operation.

Treatment could require a prostatectomy; an easy operation today. Frequently it is performed through a tiny tube inserted into the urethra.

The operation involves the removal of part of the offending gland. This is often done by a wire being passed up the tube. The end of this is activated by an electric current which disintegrates the diseased parts. In the period after the operation, plenty of fluids must be drunk (maybe ten pints or more daily). Be guided by *the doctor* on this, and do not strain when passing water or emptying the bowels.

The operation does not normally affect love-life or sex pleasure. For anatomical reasons the ejaculation of seminal fluid usually mostly or all passes into the bladder instead of as formerly. Consult with the surgeon to see if special treatment can be arranged to preserve fertility, and whether sex pleasure will be affected, then *accept his assurances,* because it is important to retain confidence. (*See* IMPOTENCE, FREQUENCY OF URINATION, RETENTION OF URINE.)

Pruritus.
Medical term for itching. A particularly distressing form of intense pruritus known as pruritus vulvae (itching and inflammation of the external parts) occurs in women and is often due to thrush. This is common in diabetes (*See* DIABETES).

Psoriasis.
A common skin disease in which hard, red, scaly patches appear. They often affect the skin near joints such as the elbows, or behind the knees, though other areas are often involved. Unfortunately the disease is a chronic one, and the patches are difficult to clear up. The exact cause is not known, but the disease is not dangerous. Sufferers often enjoy good health, although an associated arthritis may occur in some susceptible patients.

Treatment of psoriasis is a long-term problem. Local steroid, tar and dithranol ointments are often helpful. Recently a combination of tablets and special ultra-violet radiation (P.U.V.A.) has been found to help in many cases. Although the disease is nothing to do with cancer some anti-cancer drugs are also proving effective. Keep in touch with your doctor as advances may be on the way.

Psychosis.

Describes any serious mental disturbance in which the patient has little or no insight into his condition. (*See* MENTAL ILLNESS.)

FIG. 11 Taking the pulse

Pulse.

The pulse is caused by an expansion of the arteries which corresponds with each heart beat. Counting the pulse is a convenient way of counting the heartbeats. In most infectious illnesses the heart beats faster than usual and the rate of the heartbeat often provides useful information to the doctor. A very slow pulse (forty beats a minute or less) if associated with other symptoms of ill health can indicate heart block or certain other serious illnesses. The treatment may be an artificial pacemaker (*See* HEART DISEASE). Athletes and many athletic people in robust health may have a slow pulse (fifty beats a minute) and anyone with this tendency need not worry if their health is otherwise good. The pulse may be counted from any artery, but the one at the wrists is usually chosen. The radial artery runs over the bones at the front of the wrist below the base of the thumb.

To count the pulse, the finger-tips should be placed in line over the artery with the patient's wrist straight, and the beats should be counted for a minute. (*See* FIG. 11.) The normal rate for an adult is about 70 to 80 beats per minute.

Purpura.

A condition in which a rash of many small purplish red spots appears in the skin. There are several causes. It may be due to an abnormality of the blood or to a disease of the smallest blood vessels, or capillaries, which allow a little blood to leak. The spots which are tiny collections of blood – about the size of a pinhead – may also form in the internal organs. Pressure on the spots causes them to pale as the blood is pushed to one side. It is not easy to generalise about this since the course of the disease depends upon the type. Some are serious, and the patient is gravely ill, while in others the condition is merely a passing inconvenience. The mild type of purpura may sometimes accompany other infectious illnesses or may be a form of allergic response to a germ or drug.

Pus.

When a part of the body is attacked by germs a thick fluid is often formed, known as *pus*. For further information *see* ABSCESS.

Pyelonephritis *(pyelitis)*.

The human kidney can be divided into two parts. The outer layer of the organ is made up of small blood vessels and tubes into which the impurities from the blood are filtered. These tubes open into an inner chamber or small sac known as the pelvis of the kidney, in which the urine collects. Sometimes this part is attacked by germs, which usually reach it via the bladder, and this condition is known as pyelitis. As there is always some degree of spread of infection from the collecting channels to the "true" kidney the illness should really be thought of as pyelo*nephritis*. It is more common in women. (*See* CYSTITIS.) The symptoms are pain in the loin, pain and frequency in passing water and a very high temperature (105°F, 40½°C is not unusual). Sometimes there is vomiting and there may be attacks of shivering (rigors). The treatment of pyelonephritis is bed rest, plenty of fluids and appropriate antibiotics. Recurrent attacks indicate that more complete kidney investigation is called for and even one attack in a child needs specialist investigation. The long term effects of neglected pyelonephritis include kidney failure.

Pyorrhoea.

A chronic infection of the gums leading to discharge of pus and loosening of the teeth. It is not a condition which one can neglect. Not only is there danger of losing the teeth but poison from the infection is swallowed and may cause indigestion etc. The sooner your dentist can start treatment the easier it should be to cure. The disease may possibly be prevented if the gums are brushed regularly up and down when washing the teeth. In old age teeth may become loose through "wear and tear".

Pyrexia. (*See* FEVER *and* TEMPERATURE)

Q

Quarantine (*and incubation periods*).

The period of time during which a disease may develop after exposure to infection. Most diseases have an incubation period, during which, although the germs are in the body, they do not produce symptoms. In a cold, for instance, the incubation period is usually three days – it takes three days to develop after "catching" it from someone. During this period the illness is infectious although the carrier is still feeling well. Quarantine implies the shutting away of the suspect from all other contacts except necessary medical and nursing staff and immune people for a period of time equal to the incubation period plus two days. This is no longer necessary in the case of trivial or easily treated illnesses where more is lost than gained by the procedure. It is, however, vital in life-threatening illnesses like smallpox, cholera, typhoid fever and poliomyelitis where all contacts should be strictly isolated during the quarantine period.

With the common childhood illnesses, the *sufferer* is of course excluded from school for certain periods which vary with the severity of the illness and local schools' requirements. You must be guided by your doctor but in general the child requires one week at home for German measles, two weeks for chickenpox and mumps, two to three weeks for measles and at least three weeks for whooping cough. In dysentery and food poisoning the sufferer can return to work when medical testing of stool samples is found to be satisfactory. Those whose work is in any way connected with food should report to a doctor immediately with any symptoms such as nausea, vomiting, abdominal pain or loose motions.

Incubation periods for the common infections are shown:

Chicken pox	*21 days*	*Measles*	*16 days*
German measles	*22 days*	*Scarlatina*	*10 days*
Influenza	*5 days*	*(Scarlet Fever)*	
Mumps	*28 days*	*Whooping Cough*	*21 days*

Quinsy.

An abscess on the tonsil (*See* ABSCESS). The tonsil is liable to infection and sometimes this spreads beneath the tonsil where a small abscess forms. There is a fairly high temperature, considerable swelling of the throat, and pain. Penicillin is usually prescribed but sometimes the quinsy bursts releasing the pus. Occasionally it may have to be "lanced" by the doctor before it will clear up.

R

Rabies. (*See* DOG BITE)

Rash.

The name of an eruption on the skin. There are many types, all of which have special names:

Erythema a diffuse redness of the skin – like a blush. It may follow exposure to the sun or a mild burn.

Macules are small patches on the skin which are *not* raised above the surface. A freckle could be described as a brown macule. Red macules occur in certain skin diseases.

Papules are small pimples on the skin. The rash of measles usually consists of a mixture of macules and papules. Thus there is a patchy discolouration of the skin in some places *not* raised above the surface, and in other places raised into small bumps.

Vesicles are small blisters containing fluid. (They occur in chickenpox.)

Pustules are small blisters containing pus or "matter." They occur in ACNE and in many other conditions.

Raynaud's Disease.

People develop white, numb fingers if subjected to intense cold. If they occur more readily and frequently than average it is known as Raynaud's phenomenon which means that the tiny arteries carrying blood to the fingers have clamped down to prevent blood entering the extremities. Sometimes it is a symptom of a more general disorder or it can be an isolated feature. The condition can be helped by tablets which open up blood vessels. If simple tablets like Pernivit, taken one three times a day do not help it is best to seek medical advice. (*See* CHILBLAINS, FROSTBITE)

Recuperation (*after an illness or operation*).

Some illnesses leave one weak and liable to a relapse.

After illness or operation, aim at recovering slowly, but *steadily*. That is the important point.

When in bed, and especially after surgery you will be advised to keep toes, legs, etc., moving. This is to prevent stagnation and thrombosis in a deep leg vein which could lead to a blood clot reaching the lung (*See* THROMBOSIS *and* EMBOLISM). Physical exercise strengthens, provided it is used wisely, regularly, and never beyond exhaustion point. The first day up one may manage only to walk ten yards, the next day 50–100 may be possible. Do realise the speed at which returning *physical* and *mental* activity can *surge back*, even in the very old.

Avoid over-hot baths which can induce faintness. A tonic prescribed by your doctor may help but *it is the will to get well that matters*. Healing tissues need plenty of vitamin C, obtainable from oranges or vitamin mixtures like Orovite 7. Sunshine, too, is a great tonic, (as well as promoting extra vitamin D in the skin) and a convalescent holiday in the sun is recommended.

After even major operations, and illnesses such as coronary thrombosis, graduated walking exercises should get you ready for sedentary work by the six week stage. If you do manual work this may take longer – perhaps up to three months. You should also be ready to resume sexual intercourse somewhere between the six and twelve week stage. Talk to your doctor for specific advice.

After certain operations, especially abdominal ones, coughing can cause hernias so smokers are advised to give it up. Straining to open the bowels can have the same effect.

Healing of long bones may require prolonged immobilization in hospital. Here the importance of the will to get well is even more vital. One hundred per cent co-operation with prescribed exercises and physiotherapy is usually the mainstay of treatment – active exercise often being more important than passive massage, etc.

Renal Colic.

It sometimes happens that stones form within the kidney – usually in the collecting part of the kidney, or pelvis (*see* PYELONEPHRITIS). If the stone is small it may try to pass from the kidney to the bladder through a narrow tube known as the ureter. This usually causes a severe pain which comes on in spasms and is known as *renal colic*. This pain commonly starts in the loin and radiates downwards towards the groin on the same side. It may be accompanied by blood in the urine due to injury to the ureter as the stone passes through it. The condition calls for expert treatment, and is often best dealt with in hospital where X-rays and other means of investigation are available. The presence of blood in the water (HAEMATURIA) is always an indication of something amiss and should demand medical attention. (*See* CALCULUS, KIDNEY DISEASE, PROSTATE.)

Retention of Urine.

When urine has collected in the bladder the pressure rises and we feel a desire to pass water. When circumstances permit, we allow the muscle guarding the exit from the bladder to relax and it is emptied. *Retention of urine* means that there is some interference with this emptying and either the bladder cannot be emptied, (*acute retention*) or emptying is not complete. Acute retention most often occurs in elderly men due to a swelling of the prostate gland. Medical assistance must be sent for at once, and it is often essential for the doctor to pass a tube (catheter) to draw off the urine. Acute retention can occur in women during the early months of pregnancy, when, if the womb becomes displaced, it may press on the lower part of the bladder. It is usually not difficult to "replace" the womb when the condition clears. Difficulty in passing water usually precedes retention. Seek advice now and do not wait until it is serious. (*See* PREGNANCY, PROSTATE.)

Sometimes inability to pass urine is due to shyness, for example, in a public toilet or hospital. This has no physical cause and cures in time. Certain drugs can also cause this.

Retina.

The innermost of the three coats surrounding the eye; it is the part sensitive to light and which registers images.

Retinitis Pigmentosa.

A hereditary condition in which the retina becomes progressively thickened and coated with pigment (coloured material) so that vision gradually deteriorates. Research into methods of treatment continues.

Retroversion.

The tipping of an entire organ backward. The term is commonly used to describe the womb. Twenty per cent of women are born with the uterus lying in this position and unless it is giving rise to discomfort or contributing to infertility there is no need for any treatment.

Rhesus Factor.

As well as being classified into A, O, B and AB groups, blood can be divided into *rhesus positive* and *rhesus nega-*

tive types depending on the presence or absence of rhesus factors on the red blood cells. Problems used to arise when a rhesus negative mother married to a rhesus positive father gave birth to a rhesus positive baby. The mother manufactured "antibodies" to the baby's red blood cells which had crossed into her circulation through the placenta (*see* BIRTH). These antibodies could then pass back into the baby's blood through the umbilical cord and destroy his red blood cells causing jaundice and anaemia.

The danger period for the passage of baby red cells into the maternal blood is at the time of a birth or miscarriage when the placenta separates from the uterus lining. This explains why a first baby was usually unaffected (unless there had been a previous miscarriage).

A great advance in recent years has been the introduction of "Anti-Rhesus D" serum which is now given to rhesus negative mothers in the U.K. at the time of each delivery or miscarriage. This serum "mops up" any baby red cells which have got into the mother's circulation before they have had time to induce antibodies. There has thus been a great reduction in numbers of severely affected babies needing exchange blood transfusion or being damaged by jaundice.

In the U.K. mothers are routinely blood grouped and tested for antibodies at various stages of pregnancy so that "at risk" babies can be detected before birth and perhaps induced early if this seems to be in their best interests. Due to "Anti D" these premature inductions are becoming rarer.

Rheumatic Fever.

Now a relatively rare illness, but commonest in children, it usually follows a throat infection with a particular type of streptococcus germ. After an interval of about six weeks the body's fighting forces including antibodies over-react and turn on its own tissues, particularly the joints, and cause inflammation. These reactions may also involve the muscle and valves of the heart. A fever, sore throat and swollen painful joints are typical.

Occasionally the brain may become involved leading to the jerky, uncontrolled movements known as St. Vitus'

Dance (*See* CHOREA). Antibiotics, especially, penicillin, are effective in curing the original streptococcal infection and help to prevent Rheumatic Fever nowadays. Another reason for its rarity is a change in the nature of the streptococcus which has become a milder germ. If it *does* develop, treatment is bedrest to rest the joints and the heart and a prolonged course of penicillin. Other drugs such as cortisone are used to minimise joint and heart damage. Sometimes after recovery, which may take several weeks, the patient is left with a damaged heart valve. Modern surgical techniques are often effective in repairing or replacing the valves.

Rheumatism.

A vague term covering conditions associated with pain in the joints or limbs. Rheumatism which affects the joints is more accurately known as ARTHRITIS, and the reader should consult this article. Other varieties of the condition are described under MUSCULAR RHEUMATISM and BACKACHE.

Rheumatoid Arthritis. (*See* ARTHRITIS)

Rickets.

A deficiency disease, due to lack of vitamin D (*see* PAGE 10) which affects growing children. For the proper growth and strengthening of bones calcium is required, and it cannot be absorbed from the diet and utilized by the body without the aid of small quantities of vitamin D. This vitamin occurs chiefly in milk and butter, but can also be manufactured by the body with the aid of sunlight – but not without. If the diet is lacking in the vitamin-containing foods, and if the child does not receive much sunshine, then the absorption of calcium is liable to fall below the minimum requirements. When this happens growth is stunted and the bones become soft and bend. *Rickets* is rare in England because steps are taken to see that all children have adequate vitamin D. Flour, margarine and cereals usually have vitamin D added artificially and vitamin drops (Abidec) are provided at welfare clinics for the under fives. Occasionally the disease is still seen in Asian immigrants and in poorer lands.

Rigor.

An attack of shivering which occurs when the temperature is raised. When the body wishes to increase its temperature one of the ways it can do this is by shivering. This sets the muscles working in little to and fro movements, which generate heat. Normally, when the body becomes chilled shivering is liable to occur. If the body is invaded by germs and the temperature rises suddenly severe shivering attacks may occur and these are known as *rigors*. Nature at work! (*See* PYELONEPHRITIS *and* MALARIA)

Ringworm.

Caused by a fungus, or yeast-like organism, which attacks the skin and the roots of the hairs. It is contagious and may occur in epidemics, for instance in schools. It commonly affects the hairy skin at the back of the neck, and the infection spreads in a circular fashion, forming a round area which gives the disease its name. Ointments containing anti-fungal drugs are usually effective although tablets (griseofulvin) may be needed in resistant cases.

S

Salpingitis.

The top of the womb is connected by means of two small tubes, the fallopian tubes, to the ovaries, one on either side of the lower part of the abdominal cavity. When the tubes become inflamed the condition is known as *salpingitis,* which may accompany or follow any infection of the womb and vagina. One cause is neglected gonorrhoea, in which the infection gradually works its way up until the tubes are involved. Less common nowadays is tuberculous salpingitis. Salpingitis, in common with most infections, is usually accompanied by fever, and there is pain low down on either side of the abdomen. If the right tube is affected, the condition may be mistaken for appendicitis. It must not be neglected, especially as it sometimes causes sterility. Treatment is by antibiotics and radiant heat. (*See* ECTOPIC PREGNANCY, GONORRHOEA *and* INFERTILITY.)

Sarcoidosis.

A disorder which may affect many organs including the skin, glands, lungs and liver. The first signs are often purple patches on the shins known as erythema nodosum. If the lungs are involved there may be shortness of breath. Fortunately the condition responds well to steroids so unusual patches on the shins should always be mentioned to your doctor in case these are an early sign (although there are other more trivial causes).

Scabies.

A skin disease known as the "itch" and caused by a small mite. It makes small burrows in the skin where it lays its eggs; and since it is active when the skin is warm, the itching is usually at its worst in bed at night, or when sitting by the fire. The hands, particularly the webs of the fingers, and the wrists are the parts most often affected. It is contagious, being passed from one to another, and like louse infestation is favoured by overcrowding and lack of cleanliness.

Treatment consists in having a hot bath and scrubbing the affected parts with a stiff brush to open up the burrows, changing and boiling all the clothing and bedclothes, and applying something to kill the mites. One of the most effective is Benzyl Benzoate or Quellada lotion applied to the whole body from neck downwards and left for 24 hours before washing off. Two applications separated by five days nearly always cure but unless the clothes are properly dealt with, and all the members of the family and pets are cleared, re-infection is likely.

Scalds. (*See* BURNS)

Scarlet Fever.

Once a killing disease scarlet fever is less serious because the germ which causes it, a streptococcus, has become less violent. It is infectious with a short incubation period (3–5 days) starting as a sore throat, tonsillitis and fever. A skin rash appears a day or two later with a general reddening (erythema) except around the mouth area which is pale. Mild forms are often known as scarlatina. It responds rapidly to penicillin and long-term complications such as nephritis and rheumatic fever are now rare.

Schizophrenia.

Describes a seriously disordered mind, where thought and behaviour lose touch with reality, i.e. in the acute stage the sufferer is psychotic. There are several types, including the paranoid form, and sufferers may be suspicious, possibly only of some people. In the classical form, thinking becomes disjointed and the emotions and reactions inappropriate. The patient may hear "voices" giving instructions, and because of this may occasionally act dangerously. Judgement and control of emotions suffer, delusions are common, and the person can become unwilling or unable to co-operate with friends and medical advisers. He may end in collapse. The invalid is unbalanced, and his family "do not know what to do".

Anyone may display these symptoms once or twice in their life but this would not be true schizophrenia. Doctors would only diagnose schizophrenia if symptoms of this kind became a recurrent feature.

The interaction of mind on body is poorly understood. Nevertheless, counselling, psychotherapy and consideration of change in the life-style are likely to be of help, but only after the acute stage of this illness is controlled. In the early days the sufferer needs urgent medical help which may include long-term medication and occasionally E.C.T. (*See* ANXIETY STATE, DEPRESSION, E.C.T., MENTAL ILLNESS, PARANOIA.)

Sciatica.

Term for pain in the sciatic nerve, a large nerve running through the buttock and down the back of the leg. Sometimes the nerve becomes inflamed due to pressure from a slipped disc (*see* SLIPPED DISC), on its origins in the lumbar region. The bones of the spine or vertebrae are separated by a small disc of "gristle", and if one of these invertebral discs becomes displaced it may press upon an adjacent nerve root. Often sciatica is not serious and responds to simple remedies such as rest and tablets to reduce inflammation but if a disc is displaced traction and occasionally an operation may be required. See your doctor.

Scurvy.

Deficiency disease, due to lack of vitamin C (*see* PAGE 10). Vitamin C is necessary to keep the blood vessels healthy, and in its absence the small capillaries become weak and allow bleeding into the skin and gums. Vitamin C is found in fresh fruits and vegetables, of which nearly everyone can have an adequate supply. The disease is practically unknown in England, but occasionally occurs in the poor, the elderly or in "cranks" who adopt a peculiar diet which does not include vegetables.

Sea Sickness. (*See* TRAVEL SICKNESS *and* VOMITING)

Sebaceous Cyst. (*See* CYST)

Second Opinion.

The term means a second consultant opinion but most people use it to mean any specialist opinion arranged by the family doctor.

Your family doctor will have many consultant colleagues and access to a variety of specialist departments. Often he will suggest that you see a consultant if he feels it necessary. If he does not it may be because he is confident about the nature of your condition thinking you will obtain no benefit from further investigation or surgery. Occasionally it may be because you have minimised your symptoms or anxieties and implied that you feel better than you do.

If you are anxious about some symptoms tell him just how worried you are and why (e.g. a family history of some illness). Often a relation can put this over better than you and a word from one is often useful. Once they understand the reason for anxiety most doctors will arrange a consultant appointment. If this fails, put your request in writing. Some people are better at expressing themselves in this way and few doctors will refuse a written request. Although a specialist will sometimes see you privately without a letter of reference from your doctor he will often prefer you to have one. However, there is usually a way round any difficulty. It should rarely be necessary to change doctors but this is possible in extreme cases.

Septicaemia.

Implies that germs are multiplying fast in the blood and have almost overcome body defences. Fever then delirium occur and urgent appropriate antibiotic treatment is needed.

Sexually Transmitted Diseases. (S.T.D.)

SYPHILIS and GONORRHOEA apart, the most common is non-specific urethritis (*see* N.S.U.) often due to a germ, Chlamydia. Despite treatment complications can occur in eyes, joints. TRICHOMONAS and THRUSH which give vaginal discharge can spread by intercourse as can a grave form of HEPATITIS. Pubic LICE are also spread by intercourse. *There are more risks to casual sex than is supposed.*

The *herpes virus* (HSV-2) is another cause of S.T.D. Genital herpes usually causes sore blisters of the genitalia in both sexes. It is increasing, probably due to permissive attitudes and more use of *non-barrier* birth control. It can be recurrent and may affect the health of an unborn child if an attack occurs in pregnancy. It is also implicated in the development of cancer of the cervix some years after-wards. Until recently there was no satisfactory treatment but a new anti-viral drug "Acyclovir" seems effective. Vaccination is being tested, with promising results. A.I.D.S. (Acquired Immune Deficiency Syndrome) is a newly recog-nised disease, now mainly affecting male homosexuals. It lowers the body's natural defences against diseases including rare cancers and may be fatal. Possibly due to a virus, one fear is that the illness could be spread by blood transfusion.

Shaking. (*See* TREMOR)

Shingles.

A virus infection the same as in CHICKEN POX. In shingles, damage is confined to an area supplied to a nerve. The common site is the trunk, but may be face or limbs. Usually burning pain before other symptoms, followed by eruption. Small patches of skin are inflamed, on each are small spots with white tops on a strip of skin supplied by one nerve. In the trunk they follow a circle from back to front; usually lasts a few weeks, then subsides. The patient is best in bed during the acute stage, and the spots must be kept dry. Usually recovery is complete in about three weeks; but sometimes, particularly in the elderly, there is some persistent pain after the eruption has gone. Soothing lotions such as calamine can be helpful and an anti-virus agent "Herpid" available only on prescription if started early may reduce the severity of the pain and inflammation. The depression and debility which sometimes follow shingles may be helped by vitamin B$_{12}$. Elderly people sometimes are helped by special painkilling tablets for persistent post-shingles pain. Susceptible subjects can catch chicken pox from people with shingles and possibly vice versa.

Shock.

Medically this term means collapse of the circulation, when the blood pressure is low and the flow of blood through the tissues is reduced. It occurs most commonly after blood loss or with severe pain. The pulse becomes fast and weak, the skin pale and clammy and the breathing shallow or laboured. It requires urgent medical attention. If the patient is injured do not move him; keep him calm, ensure that breathing is unrestricted by tight clothes and keep him warmly wrapped in a blanket until medical help arrives.

Sickness. (See TRAVEL SICKNESS and VOMITING)

Sinus.

A hollow cavity often taken to mean one of the hollows in the facial bones communicating with the nose. (See ANTRUM.)

Sinusitis. (See ANTRUM)

Sleep. (See PAGE 12 and INSOMNIA)

Slipped Disc.

The spine consists of a column of strong bones (vertebrae) separated by tough but compressible "discs". Occasionally a disc, which is rather like a cushion, becomes damaged and its gelatinous "stuffing" is squeezed out by the pressure from the vertebrae. This causes pressure on surrounding tissues and the result is severe back pain.

When the nerves emerging from the spinal cord are compressed the result is sciatica, pain in the buttock and leg. Tingling or numbness in the calf or foot often follows. A slipped disc can be treated in many ways. Bed rest, a supporting plaster or corset, and traction (to pull the vertebrae steadily off the protruding disc) are often used. Relief of pain is probably due to shrivelling up of the extruded matter rather than its returning back to the disc shell.

Back strengthening exercises (*see* BACKACHE) are useful after the pain has subsided. The value of a plaster or surgical corset is that the spine can be rested while the patient continues to be up and about. Although uncomfortable this is usually preferable to a long time in bed. Occasionally, severe cases benefit from an operation in which the damaged disc is removed (laminectomy).

As the disc nucleus is made of soft gelatinous material it is unlikely in most cases that it can be "put back". More likely manipulation stretches and tears a few pieces of fibrous tissue allowing the disc to settle down into a more comfortable area with less pressure on a nerve. Everyone should aim to put as little cruel stress on the vertebral column as possible by always bending the knees to pick any item off the floor. The majority of slipped discs respond to the conservative measures outlined above plus common sense in everyday life.

All acute backache is not slipped disc. There are probably all sorts of minor displacements between the many facets of vertebrae. There is every degree of back problem ranging from the minor nuisance variety to the completely paralysing when the muscle of the thigh wastes away. Some neurotics hide behind a "bad back" but that is a different problem.

Smallpox.

Infectious illness due to a virus. Smallpox resembles chicken pox in many respects, but is a more serious illness which carries a considerable death rate. The only source of smallpox now is research laboratories since this once worldwide disease has been eradicated. Infants are no longer vaccinated routinely.

Snakebite.

Unless hospital treatment by anti-venom cannot be obtained fairly quickly it is better to do nothing except allay anxiety. Get the patient to hospital as soon as possible, and take the killed snake along for identification. If a very long delay is anticipated a broad, flat firm compress may be applied but on no account should a narrow, constricting band be used as its release may cause sudden flooding of the system with poison.

Spina Bifida.

A defect in the closure of the bony cages of the spinal cord at the time of its development before birth. Thus there may be protrusion of nervous tissue or its covering usually at a low level on the baby's back. In the least affected cases the skin is intact, only the bony cage being defective; in such types there may be no nerve damage and the condition may simply be noted by chance on X-ray.

Where there is considerable exposure of nervous tissue the patient has paralysis and loss of sensation in the pelvis and legs, including loss of control of bladder and bowel. In milder cases there is a variable degree of weakness and sensation loss.

Where possible the defect is closed surgically soon after birth but such children need intensive orthopaedic and neurological supervision to make the best use of existing faculties and to prevent muscles from contracting into a fixed, bent position. Closure of the gap may predispose to the build up of fluid circulating through the spinal canal and can cause hydrocephalus (enlargement of the head due to increased fluid in the cerebral canal) but this problem has been largely overcome by the development of a one way valve inserted near the ear to connect the brain cavity with the blood circulation. Mothers who have had one such baby or where there is a family history of the condition can have a test performed on the womb fluid at the sixteenth week of any subsequent pregnancy. The presence of a certain protein in the fluid indicates the likelihood that the baby does have a spinal defect and the mother is offered termination of pregnancy if she wishes.

A more simple blood test is now being performed on

pregnant women in some centres in the U.K. and it is expected that this will become routine here in the near future. In this way it is hoped that this sad condition will be drastically reduced.

Spleen.

The spleen lies in the upper part of the abdominal cavity on the left, under the lowest ribs. It stores blood corpuscles and releases these into the circulation if they are required in an emergency. It also removes the old, worn-out blood cells from circulation. The spleen, if badly injured, can be removed without any apparent ill effects.

FIG. 12   Bandaging a sprain

Sprains.

Joints are held together by tough bands of tissue known as ligaments. If a joint is carried beyond its normal range of movement, by a sudden twist, for instance, the ligaments binding it may be strained or torn. This is known as a *sprain*.

There is pain in the joint which persists, and soon the joint becomes swollen and stiff. One of the common joints to be sprained is the ankle, which is usually turned under while walking or running on a rough surface. The best initial treatment is a cold compress which helps to reduce the swelling. A day or two's rest is usually needed but activity can then be resumed provided that the joint has support. An elastic bandage or arthro-pad is useful; the former should be applied in a figure of eight around the foot and lower end of the leg (FIG. 12, *page* 202). It should be worn until the tenderness and swelling have gone in possibly a few days to a fortnight. The wrist too is often sprained, and it should be supported in the same way with a spiral bandage applied from the knuckles to about half way to the elbow. Consult a doctor for serious sprains, for there may be injury to the bone, in addition to the ligament injury.

Sprue. (*Coeliac Disease*)

Occurs when absorption of food from the intestines is interfered with for some reason. The patient loses weight, may become anaemic and has loose motions which have a fatty appearance. The usual cause in the U.K. is Coeliac Disease in which sensitivity to gluten can damage the delicate intestinal lining. A gluten-free diet restores normality.

Tropical sprue occurs when some form of infection leaves the intestinal lining damaged and unable to absorb food adequately. Medical investigation is required in a specialist centre.

Sputum.

Matter which is coughed up. Normally there should be none, for although there is a slight secretion within the bronchi, or breathing tubes, it does not collect sufficiently to come up on coughing. The production of sputum is an indication that the bronchi are irritated. It often occurs in heavy smokers who inhale – when the sputum is dark in colour. Sputum is also produced in a number of diseases. Bronchitis, pneumonia and tuberculosis are examples. Any persistent cough (three weeks or more) with which sputum is produced should be taken as a warning that a medical overhaul is advisable.

Squint.

Normally the eyes are co-ordinated so they point in the same direction. This enables the brain to make one picture from the images received from the separate eyes. When there is a squint (strabismus) the eye muscles are out of balance so that one eye points inwards or outwards. This makes it difficult for the brain to fuse the two images, so that after a time the affected eye becomes "lazy" and takes little part in vision. It is important that a squint should be treated early before the affected eye has grown lazy. Squinting is only normal in the first few weeks of life and if neglected the eye will eventually become sightless. If it persists after three months seek advice. Treatment may be by a combination of exercises, covering the sound eye for a time in order to make the squinting eye do more work, by prescribing glasses, and sometimes operation to improve the cosmetic effect.

St. Vitus' Dance. (*See* CHOREA)

Stammering.

Speech defect in which there is a recurrent hesitation in the flow of words. There are different types of stammering, one of the most common being a repetition of the beginning of a word, especially if it begins with a consonant (e.g. c-c-c-c-consonant). The condition is always made worse by nervousness, which often sets up a vicious circle, the patient being afraid that he will stammer and therefore stammering more. Seek expert treatment for a young child who stammers. Special methods of speech-therapy have been developed, and it is easier to cure the abnormality before it is firmly established. Ask your local Child Clinic (in the U.K.) if you are anxious in any way about your four year old child's speech. Hearing may need to be checked and if speech therapy does prove to be necessary this will allow plenty of time before starting school. Although many minor defects at this stage are simply due to immaturity it is better to be certain both about hearing acuity and speech.

Stings.

Insects, bees, wasps and ants, etc., are able to injure tissues by injecting material by means of a special sting or biting. The material which produces the irritation is usually an acid, and the pain can sometimes be alleviated by applying an alkali. This may be done by using a wet compress on which sodium bicarbonate has been sprinkled. One exception is the wasp which produces an alkaline sting so that an application of vinegar may be soothing. Wasps almost never sting, if you leave them alone. It is the honey bee that is vicious, especially in bad weather. An antihistamine cream such as Anthisan is probably the most helpful for any sting but should not be used more than four times daily for three days as allergy to the cream can develop. Stings are usually not serious, but scratching should be avoided since it may introduce germs and so lead to infection. Be wary to watch every bite when out picnicking. Wasp stings on the tongue are dangerous leading to swelling which can cause breathing difficulties. Urgent medical attention is necessary.

It is possible to become allergic to insect stings and if your skin reaction seems to be excessive consult your doctor so as to avoid future trouble. In extreme allergic reactions there may be swelling of the throat causing breathing difficulties and collapse of the circulation. You should have antihistamine tablets (e.g. piriton) with you if you are allergic to bee stings, but probably the best emergency treatment for allergy to bee stings is the use of an adrenaline inhaler "Medihaler Epi". One to three puffs should be taken immediately and can be repeated in thirty minutes. This inhaler was originally designed as an asthma treatment but is quicker and more effective than the injections previously recommended for severe sting allergy. In the U.K. ask your doctor about this as a prescription is needed.

Insect repellant creams which are not unpleasant to use can be purchased at all chemists' shops and these may reduce insect attacks. Some people find that taking vitamin B and C tablets such as "BC 500" or "Allbee with C" wards off attacks.

Stones. *(See* CALCULUS, RENAL COLIC *and* GALL BLADDER*)*

Stroke.

Broadly speaking, the right half of the body is controlled by the left half of the brain and vice versa. A stroke often causes a weakness of one half of the body. It is due to damage to the opposite half of the brain, and nearly always results from some interference with the blood supply. One of the causes is a *cerebral* haemorrhage in which there is bleeding into the tissues of the brain due to a rupture of a blood vessel. This is sometimes a late consequence of untreated high blood pressure, or may be due to a weak patch in one of the arteries in the brain. In other cases the stroke is not due to bleeding but to a blood clot in one of the arteries, which deprives a part of the brain of its blood. Sometimes the clot forms in the vessel due perhaps to a rough patch on the wall. This is a *cerebral thrombosis.* Or the clot may form elsewhere and be carried to the brain in the circulation, plugging one of the arteries – a *cerebral embolism.*

Whatever the cause the results are similar. The patient may become unconscious, one half of the body may be found to be weakened and there may be loss of speech. Often much smaller strokes occur in which there may be only slight weakness of one limb or slurring of speech.

Recovery is often complete and rapid perhaps within a day or two. These very small strokes are often referred to as "spasms", the assumption being that a blood vessel has closed up – then opened again. "Spasms" are a useful warning as they often allow some risk factor such as high blood pressure to be recognised and treated. Even with larger strokes there is often a considerable recovery, since the remaining undamaged parts of the brain are able to take over many of the functions of the damaged part. This takes time and calls for perseverance by the patient. Usually the younger the victim the more the recovery that can be expected, and anyone who has suffered from a stroke must never give up hope.

Physiotherapy can be arranged and if exercises are carried out regularly, slow but steady improvement will usually reward the victim. A useful exercise for a weak hand is to squeeze a soft ball (or plastic pan scourer) twenty times four times a day. Speech therapy is helpful for those whose speech is affected and this may also include retraining in handwriting. The local Social Service Departments (in the U.K.) are very helpful in suggesting and fitting devices in the home to make daily living easier for a stroke victim. Your family doctor can put you in touch with the various agencies who are able to help.

Stye.

A small boil which develops on the eyelid due to infection at the root of one of the eyelashes. It usually clears spontaneously but may be helped by using an antiseptic eye ointment such as Brolene. Recurrent styes may indicate the need for an antibiotic eye ointment and medical investigation into general health. A course of vitamin B tablets such as Becosym may help to prevent recurrences.

Suffocation.

Occurs when the body is deprived of air for some reason. (*See* ASPHYXIA *and* ARTIFICIAL RESPIRATION.)

Sulphonamides.

These drugs were discovered originally during research into chemical dyes; they combat bacterial infections in a similar way to antibiotics. M & B was one of the earliest to be in common use in the U.K. Except in infections of the bladder and kidneys sulphonamides have been largely superseded by ANTIBIOTICS, especially penicillin.

Sunburn.

After exposure to sun the skin produces a brown pigment which helps to protect it from damage by ultra-violet rays. The development of a "tan" takes time, and if the skin is exposed for too long before this has occurred, it may be severely burnt. *The symptoms are delayed*, so the fact one feels comfortable while sunbathing is no guarantee that damage is not being done. People vary in their sensitivity, fair and redheads usually being more sensitive than the dark. Take special care when coming into contact with strong sunlight for the first time after winter. Five minutes sunbathing is probably more than enough on the first day and this may be increased daily if there is no soreness. If the skin has become burnt all exposure must be stopped until the burn subsides. Remember that while oiling the skin may keep it supple and help towards an even tan, the oil will *not necessarily protect* against sunburn. Suntan creams are more suitable than oil for the fairskinned and for those who cannot tolerate sunlight at all, preparations such as Uvistat or Spectraban are helpful; these latter are almost totally impervious to sunlight. Remember also that the time spent bathing must be counted in the time of exposure since ultra-violet rays penetrate some distance in water. If you do get burned a useful cream, which can be obtained from the chemist, is caladryl; but this must be kept out of the eyes and mouth.

Sunstroke.

Due to over-exposure to the sun especially of head and neck, and caused by overheating. Sunlight is rich in infra-red rays which cause heating of the body tissues. Prolonged exposure without any head and neck covering is liable to be followed by severe headache and general prostration. Prevention is easy. No one should remain long in strong sun without adequate cover, preferably of light colour which must also shade the back of the neck. The headache which results in the unwary can usually be relieved by soluble aspirins, and for severe cases a day in bed following the exposure will usually cure. In hot climates extra salt is required with food in order to replace that lost by excessive sweating.

Suppuration. (*Festering*) (*See* ABSCESS)

Syphilis.

Most serious of the venereal diseases – i.e. diseases spread by sexual contact, due to a specific germ, a spirochaete. The disease can be divided into well-marked stages. The incubation period is usually four to five weeks but may vary between 10 and 90 days. The first symptoms (primary stage) is a small painless spot at the site of infection, usually the genitals, but very occasionally elsewhere such as the lips. This spot breaks down into an ulcer or small sore, oozing serum which is highly infective; and the glands in the neighbourhood often become a little swollen. The severity of this sore, or *chancre,* is variable; and it may be small and only temporary. It is liable to be missed especially in women because of its internal situation. Because of this any young person who has indulged in casual sex relations should be checked in a V.D. (special) clinic even if there are vague symptoms or no symptoms at all. The use of barrier methods of contraception such as cap or sheath give some protection against syphilis but the contraceptive pill gives no protection. In a totally steady sexual relationship where each partner is faithful to the other and each has no history of infection there is, of course, no risk of venereal disease. Where sex is taken casually there is always danger of infection and if worried it is wise to put your mind at rest by clinic checks. It is also a good idea to make sure that the man always uses a sheath.

Lists of venereal disease clinics in the U.K. can be found in the telephone directory and all treatment and advice is secret. As the long term effects of syphilis are so dangerous it is vital that sexual contacts are traced and clinic staff help in this task. Patients are obviously told to refrain from sexual relations until treatment is completed. Occasionally patients will not comply with this but at least they can make sure that a sheath is worn.

From the site of infection the spirochaete passes into the blood and is distributed throughout the body. This is the secondary stage. Usually there is a generalized rash which develops three or four weeks after the chancre, and the glands in other parts of the body may enlarge. The rash takes different forms, and may be associated with ulcers in the mouth and some falling of the hair. From the second stage the disease passes into the third, in which deep, painless ulcers, known as gummata, may form in various internal organs and skin. In the late stages the nervous system is particularly liable to be attacked. There may be a slow paralysis in which walking becomes more and more unsteady due to degeneration of the spinal cord known as *tabes dorsalis*; or in other cases the brain is affected, and there is a generalized paralysis together with progressive mental impairment – a condition known as *general paralysis of the insane* (G.P.I.). Practically no organ in the body is immune in the late stages of untreated syphilis. The heart may be damaged, the liver affected and vision lost. The course of the disease is slow, and symptoms involving the nervous system may develop twenty or more years after the original infection. The disease is practically never caught apart from sexual union, since the spirochaete dies rapidly outside the human body; infection from a lavatory seat is very unlikely. Infection through kissing is rare although chancres on the lip can be contacted by orogenital sexual acts. Syphilis can be passed to the unborn child of an infected mother but this condition is now rare. All pregnant women in U.K. are tested for the diease at their first antenatal hospital appointment.

Syphilis can be cured. Early treatment is essential. It cannot be too strongly emphasized that the disease is insidious, and any suspicious symptoms in anyone who has run a danger of infection should lead to advice being sought. Penicillin is a powerful weapon in the fight against syphilis but treatment must be completed. Even though all the symptoms have disappeared, and you feel perfectly well, the germs may still be lurking in part of the body, and can produce their effects years later. It is therefore dangerous and extremely foolish to stop treatment before your doctor is satisfied that it has been sufficient. Even then he will almost certainly ask you to report back after an interval for further tests. For your own sake and for the sake of those you might infect it is vital that you should do this.

There is no real prevention against syphilis except the avoidance of casual sex; the promiscuous will always run into danger of infection.

T

Tachycardia.

Term for an increased heart rate. This commonly occurs when the temperature is raised (*See* PULSE); or with a normal temperature may be due to nervousness when it is associated with palpitations. It is occasionally due to heart disease, and another not uncommon cause is an over-action of the thyroid gland. (*See* GOITRE, PALPITATIONS)

Talipes (*Clubfoot*).

A deformity of the foot, present at birth, in which the foot is twisted and fixed inwards or out. The more serious is known as equinovarus where the heel is turned inwards from the midline of the leg and the foot is bent under. In mild cases massage and splinting may suffice to straighten the foot. For serious types operation is needed to divide the ligaments which are holding the foot abnormally. Due to careful orthopaedic surgery, most of these youngsters end up with near-perfect feet and the ugly old condition of clubfoot is disappearing.

Temperature.

Temperature — How to take it

1. Hold the thermometer between the finger and thumb at the top end, away from the bulb.

FIG. 13 The thermometer
Showing both Fahrenheit and Centigrade

2. Stand facing the light and hold the thermometer horizontally a little below the eyes. Find the markings and figures which show the level of the temperature.
3. Roll the thermometer slightly backwards and forwards between finger and thumb. The light will be reflected from the mercury in the small central tube.
4. If the mercury is up in the stem of the thermometer shake it down into the bulb with a few vigorous jerks.
5. Look again and make quite sure that the mercury is down. Place the thermometer bulb well inside the mouth beneath the tongue, or, in the case of a child, in the armpit while holding the arm to the side.
6. Leave the thermometer in the mouth for at least a full minute, or beneath the arm for two minutes.

7. Hold the thermometer to the light again, turn it to reflect the mercury and find the level as described above (3).

8. Compare the mercury with the readings. The degrees are marked by numbers – 97°, 102°, etc., Fahrenheit or 37°, 38°, etc., Centigrade, known sometimes as Celsius. Some thermometers show dual scales. Between each number are marked ten small divisions. Find the number next below the mercury level and then count up the small divisions until the level is reached. This gives the temperature. Thus if the mercury is three divisions above 99° the temperature is 99·3 (ninety-nine point three). In most thermometers the normal temperature level (98·4) is marked by a small arrow, while in Centigrade normal is approximately 37°. After using the thermometer, do *not* wash it in hot water as it will burst.

Tennis Elbow.

Caused by strain of the muscles which straighten the arm at the elbow. Rarely caused by tennis, it often follows activities like house painting where the strain is more sustained. The arm needs rest for up to three weeks. An arthro-pad worn for a day or two will often speed recovery. One or two injections of hydrocortisone and local anaesthetic into the tender spots, if required, will usually cure. The pain may feel worse for 24 hours after the injection before improving. Heat and manipulation may be useful in stubborn cases and, rarely, a small operation is needed.

Tenosynovitis.

The tendons or leaders at the back of the hand and arm which move the fingers and wrist are encased in sheaths. The inner parts of these sheaths can become inflamed due to over-strain causing pain and a crackling sound on movement. The condition is common in young adults where work demands excessive movement of the wrist and hand. It is also common in gardeners. The wrist should be immobilized in plaster or a plaster adhesive bandage for three weeks and excessive use of the fingers and thumb avoided for two months.

Testicle. (*See* ORCHITIS. UNDESCENDED TESTICLE, VARICOCELE)

Test Tube Baby. (*See* INFERTILITY)

Tetanus. (*See* IMMUNIZATION)

This disease, known as lockjaw, is due to a specific germ. The poison from the tetanus bacillus has an action on the cells of the nervous system – which send the messages to move muscles. It causes irritability in these cells which results in a spasm, or painful contraction of the muscles. The jaw muscles may be involved, hence the name. The germ may gain entry to the body through a dog bite or dirty cut, since the germ lives in soil. After a variable interval fever and spasms begin to develop.

Tetanus is dangerous and requires intensive hospital treatment. Serum, containing antitoxin which neutralizes the poison, is of value if given early. See your doctor promptly after a dirty cut especially injury from a garden fork.

Tetanus can be prevented by immunisation with a material called toxoid. In the U.K. this is routinely given to children as triple vaccine in the first year of life. Immunity following these jabs usually lasts for seven to eight years so periodic booster injections are given during the school years and are advised for those who work on the land, with animals or in "dirty" occupations. Hospital casualty departments give routine doses of tetanus toxoid to anyone attending with cuts or grazes. Patients are then recommended to complete the course by having two more injections at six weeks and six month intervals. They should take this advice seriously. Horse serum which used to be given and which caused many allergic reactions is no longer used in the U.K.

Thermometer. (*See* TEMPERATURE)

Thrombosis.

The formation of a blood clot within a blood vessel. Normally this never occurs, but when a vessel is injured or diseased clotting sometimes takes place. Any part of the body may be the site of a thrombosis, and the symptoms will depend on the organ involved. If the clot is carried by the blood to some other site it is known as an embolus. Common danger sites for thrombosis are in the coronary arteries (*See* HEART DISEASE) and the *deep* veins in the calf. (Thrombosis of the cerebral arteries tends to occur only in the old.)

There is a slightly increased risk of thrombosis for older women on the pill and a much increased risk if then one smokes. Women waiting for a planned operation should give up the pill for six weeks before and stop smoking.

Thrombosis in the deep veins of the calf and thigh should not be confused with minor problems in superficial varicose veins (*See* VARICOSE VEINS.) The former tends to occur after surgery or childbirth if there is prolonged immobilization in bed. Stagnation of the blood in these veins can lead to thrombosis and the formation of emboli which travel to the lungs (*See* EMBOLISM). The leg is swollen and bending upwards of the foot is acutely painful. Nowadays the early mobilization after surgery and childbirth prevents many of these complications.

The thrombosed vein usually gradually opens up and other blood channels enlarge so that any leg swelling slowly subsides. Tablets to reduce clotting are given for six to twelve weeks to prevent emboli. A supporting bandage is applied to the leg and the patient is mobilized as soon as possible. Whilst on anti-coagulant tablets the patient needs regular blood tests to check that the clotting factors are staying at an acceptable level. Patients who have had a coronary thrombosis are not normally given anti-coagulant tablets as these seem to be more effective in their action on veins than on arteries. As thrombosis interferes with the normal circulation to an organ, treatment aims at care for the damaged area until recovery, whilst preventing further clots. Urgent medical advice is always needed.

Thyrotoxicosis.

Due to over-action of the thyroid gland. (*See* GOITRE)

Tic.

Spasmodic twitching of the face or eyelids. It may be hereditary or accompany disorders of the nervous system but generally it indicates stress. Cure depends on elimination of the causes of tension.

Tinea.

Name of many fungus infections of the skin. Tinea cruris is commoner in men and causes inflamed itchy patches of skin in the groins and inner aspects of the thighs. Tinea pedis is another name for ATHLETE'S FOOT. Tinea capitis and Tinea corporis are other names for RINGWORM. These conditions are spread by the use of communal towels, bath mats, etc. These practices should be avoided as fungi thrive in slightly damp areas. Creams such as Canesten and Tinaderm used twice daily for several weeks should cure. This routine should be followed by liberal dusting with powder such as Tinaderm or Mycota.

Tinnitus.

A noise in the ears such as ringing, buzzing or roaring. Some noises in the ears may be due to a remediable cause such as catarrh, middle ear infection or wax when they will disappear on removal of the cause. A pulsating sound in the ear may occur with high blood pressure which can be treated. Tinnitus proper, disorder of the nerve of hearing, cannot be cured except occasionally where there is a removable nerve tumour; it may be helped by tablets such as Stemetil. *True tinnitus always signifies some permanent hearing loss and is unfortunately becoming prevalent among youngsters in the pop scene due to prolonged exposure to loud noise.* When combined with giddiness and deafness the condition is known as Menières disease. Symptoms may be alleviated by Serc or Stemetil. (*See* DEAFNESS, GIDDINESS)

Tongue.

Inspection of the tongue is not the ritual it was as there are likely to be other important areas to be examined. Generally, in the healthy non-smoker it is clean and moist and covered in small raised areas – the papillae. "Invisible" tastebuds are widespread over the tongue and soft palate. If you are feeling well, do not look at your tongue for signs of blemishes. A small coating (brown in smokers) can appear in the healthiest now and then. The tongue will tend to be furred in any feverish condition. Antibiotics may cause a "dark" tongue due to fungus infection which can be cleared by anti-fungus lozenges. Persistent furring can sometimes be removed by fresh pineapple juice. Brushing with a soft toothbrush helps. A smooth, sore tongue can be a sign of anaemia and the tongue can be the site of infection, ulcer or tumour.

Most afflictions of the tongue are fairly obvious and it is rarely wise to be a tongue-watcher, except in the Biblical sense of its being "an unruly member!"

Tonic.

Given to stimulate the appetite, often incorporating vit-amins to give optimum nourishment after an illness.

Tonsillitis.

The tonsils are two small tissues on either side of the back of the throat (*See* FIG. 14). They are part of the lymphatic

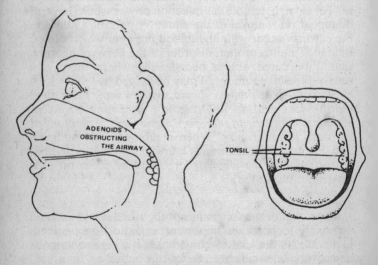

FIG. 14   Tonsils and adenoids

gland system (*See* GLAND), and trap germs which enter through the mouth. Naturally they are frequently attacked themselves, the resulting inflammation being *tonsillitis*. The first symptom is a sore throat, and if this is examined it will be seen to be inflamed. The temperature rises, the patient feels unwell, and often has a headache. As the condition progresses, the tonsils become swollen; and often can be seen to have little beads of pus, (white spots), on them. The patient should see a doctor promptly as he may need penicillin. Recurrent attacks of tonsillitis and persistently enlarged neck glands suggest that the tonsils are no longer working and may be best removed. (*See* ADENOIDS)

Toothache.

Usually due to decay which causes a cavity in a tooth or an abscess around it. See your dentist without delay; but sometimes delay is unavoidable and temporary relief required. It is difficult to suppress toothache, but one of the following may help. Soluble aspirin taken in a little water. The mouth should be rinsed with water, hot as one can bear and this swilled around the aching area. Alcohol can bring relief. A piece of cotton wool soaked in neat whisky can be applied to the tooth. Clove oil is often effective, and used in the same way. A pinch of table salt laid on the tooth is worth trying. Avoid cold food or drink. Do not bite on the affected tooth until it has been treated.

Tooth decay is due to many factors but the most important is diet. A diet rich in sugar and soft foods leads to rotten teeth so avoid excess of these. Sweets should not be eaten between meals. If eaten at the end of a meal make sure the teeth are cleaned afterwards. Teeth should be cleaned twice a day preferably with a fluoride-containing toothpaste. If you live in an area with low fluoride levels in the tap water, children's teeth can be strengthened by giving fluoride tablets (from chemist's) during the years of growth. Habits are acquired when young so make sure children use their own toothbrushes. A six monthly check with your dentist is essential to catch any possible trouble early. Meanwhile, the use of dental floss helps to remove dental plaque (where the rot starts).

Torsion of Testis.

The twisting of a testicle on its stalk leading to strangulation of the blood supply and risk of severe tissue damage if not restored rapidly to a normal position. The signs may resemble orchitis, i.e. swelling and acute pain; often vomiting occurs. Any male (often a boy) with these symptoms needs urgent medical assessment as a small operation is needed as soon as possible to prevent degeneration of the testicle. (*See* ORCHITIS)

Toxin.

Medical name for a poison produced by a germ. The toxins of diphtheria and tetanus are responsible for all the symptoms of the diseases. When invaded by germs the body can produce an *anti-toxin* which will neutralize the toxin. The basis of serum treatment, used in a number of diseases, is to supply the correct anti-toxin artificially.

Train Sickness. (*See* TRAVEL SICKNESS)

Transplants.

Transplantation surgery is a modern technique by which certain organs can be transferred to patients with severely diseased ones. With kidneys, a living donor, usually a close relative with "matching" tissue can be used, and the operations to remove one kidney from the donor and transfer it to the patient are performed simultaneously. In the case of liver, heart and in other kidney transplantations the organs of fatal accident victims are usually used. This is because at the time of death the organs are generally not affected by disease. An exception is the cornea (transparent membrane at the front of the eye). It is often of value at whatever age the donor died.

Apart from the cornea, which can restore sight to those afflicted with a disease causing clouding in this transparent membrane, the most successful transplants are kidney. Many thousands of people are alive and well because of a kidney transplant. They usually feel fitter than when dependent on a kidney machine. To prevent the body rejecting the "foreign" organ special drugs need to be taken. There is always a shortage of suitable donor kidneys.

Kidney donor cards available from doctors' surgeries, health clinics and hospitals should be carried by anyone who wishes his kidneys to be used for transplant after his death. People who wish to donate their eyes (corneas) after death should contact the Secretary General of the Royal National Institute for the Blind for details.

Travel Sickness.

The ear is an organ of balance as well as of hearing (*See* GIDDINESS). When the balancing mechanism is overstimulated it may set up a reflex (*See* PAIN) within the brain which causes vomiting. This is the basis of travel sickness which is due to constant motion, and the mechanism is the same whether it be sea, air, (*See* EARACHE) car or train sickness. Some people are better able to stand movement than others; but in everyone the balancing mechanism can gradually adjust itself, so that after some days the tendency to sickness wears off. The worst time is at the beginning of a journey, and it is then that precautions are most required.

It is best not to load the stomach, and only a light meal should be taken before embarking by those who are prone to sickness. Tablets such as Avomine which can be obtained at the chemists may help. For adults – one tablet is taken half an hour before the journey and may be repeated four hourly. Children aged six to twelve take half the adult dose. For younger children ask your doctor's advice. Looking down seems to upset the vomiting reflex so reading, especially in a car, is not advisable. Taking an interest in the surrounding scenery and having an occasional barley sugar sweet is beneficial. (*See* VOMITING)

Tremor. (*Shaking*)

Means involuntary shaking of hands or other parts due to some imbalance of the muscle and nerve action. Some people are born with naturally rather unsteady hands and this is generally of no significance. Most people become rather tremulous when nervous and again this is the normal response to fear. With increasing age it is usual for the hands to be less steady than in youth.

If tremor is of fairly sudden onset, is present at all times without obvious reason, or is causing accidents, see a doctor as it could be a symptom of remediable illnesses such as thyrotoxicosis (*See* GOITRE).

Tuberculosis.

Is caused by a specific germ – the tubercle bacillus. It lives within a special protecting membrane, and is difficult to kill, so that the infection is usually long and drawn out. Any part of the body may be attacked, but the common site is in the lungs, *pulmonary tuberculosis*. Germs are spread by persons who have the disease, and after being breathed in, they settle in the lung and multiply. Tuberculosis causes a breaking down of the normal lung tissue, so that cavities may form.

Occasionally the disease may occur in other sites such as bones, kidney and Fallopian tubes. However it responds to modern anti-tuberculous antibiotics and is now mercifully uncommon in the U.K. Hospital admission is not always necessary. Anti-tuberculous drugs need to be taken for many months but the patient can be at home for much of the time.

The infrequency of the disease in the U.K. is predominately due to public health measures, mass X-ray screening, improved nutrition, housing and effective drugs. There is also a vaccine called B.C.G. which is usually given to school children at thirteen after a skin test (Mantoux). If the skin test is negative this means that the child is not immune to tuberculosis and the vaccine is given. A positive skin test usually means that the child has met the tubercle germ already but fought it off. A chest X-ray is arranged to check that there is no disease. When tuberculosis was common this type of "natural" immunity was frequent.

There has been a recent slight increase in the incidence of tuberculosis in the U.K., especially in areas with large Asian immigrant populations. Anyone with a cough persisting for more than three weeks should go along for a chest X-Ray at the nearest centre.

Tumour.

A swelling. People become alarmed if they hear of a tumour, since tumours are a common symptom of cancer.

The word simply means "lump", and many tumours are unrelated to cancer.

Typhoid Fever. (*Enteric Fever*).

An infection of the intestines with the typhoid group of germs. Symptoms are similar to dysentery (*See* DYSENTERY), although *constipation* may be an early symptom along with fever, before a rash, abdominal pain and diarrhoea appear. The disease is more serious than dysentery but responds well to antibiotics like chloramphenicol or ampicillin. T.A.B. inoculation protects to a large degree against typhoid and similar fevers and should be given to those travelling *outside* Northern Europe, Northern America, Australia or New Zealand. The disease is spread by contaminated water and food and has been largely eliminated in the U.K. by public health measures.

U

Ulcer.

The breaking down of skin or membrane to form an open sore which may become inflamed or infected. Treatment depends on the type. Recurrent small ulcers in the mouth can be helped by putting Corlan pellets on them, or alum, and extra vitamin B, e.g. Multivite tablets. (*See* DUODENAL ULCER, GASTRIC ULCER, VARICOSE VEINS, X-RAYS)

Ultrasound.

A form of radiant energy now often used in pregnancy to determine the maturity or size of the unborn baby without using potentially harmful X-rays.

It is also used in the treatment of painful muscular or ligament disorders along with other forms of physiotherapy, heat, massage, etc.

Ultraviolet.

A form of radiant energy beyond the violet end of the spectrum; it is useful in skin disorders such as acne. As part of natural solar energy it enables the skin to produce its own natural vitamin D – responsible for strong bones and teeth.

Undescended Testicle.

The testicle normally lies within the abdominal cavity before birth. By the time the baby is born it should have moved down to occupy its position within a special sac of skin, the scrotum. Sometimes one or both organs fail to do this, and the condition is then known as an undescended testicle. Unless it occupies its normal position it cannot function properly. Sometimes it can be made to descend by means of hormone injections, but often a small operation is necessary. Remember that in small boys the testicles can retract up out of the scrotum – especially if examined with cold hands! Parents can check that the scrotum contains two small oval firm lumps at bathtime when everything is warm. Some specialists like to treat youngsters with undescended testicles at the age of four or five (others prefer to wait longer to see if natural descent will occur). If a mother suspects this condition in her four year old she should see her doctor.

Uraemia.

It occurs when the kidneys are no longer capable of filtering the poisonous waste products from the blood. There are many treatments for kidney failure ranging from low protein diet to artificial kidney machines and of course kidney transplants.

Urticaria. (*See* NETTLERASH)

Uterus. (*See* WOMB)

V

Vaccination.

Procedure used to protect against SMALLPOX by introducing germs called vaccinia into the body – now generally applied to all IMMUNIZATION.

Vagina.

The female passage. Its entrance lies between the bladder and bowel outlets. (*See* FIG. 8, *page* 103.) The opening is flanked by the two pairs of skin folds known as the labia majora and minora. The labia minora meet some way in front of the vaginal entrance and partially cover the sensitive clitoris.

Vaginismus. (*See* FRIGIDITY)

Vaginitis. (*Leucorrhoea*)

Inflammation of the vagina causing itching, soreness, painful intercourse and discharge which may be blood stained. This can occur in the absence of infection after the menopause when it is due to the lining becoming thinner and less resilient as oestrogen levels decline. This type of vaginitis may be helped by oestrogen cream but your doctor's advice is essential first. This vaginitis may go on to become infected by germs and may be associated with troublesome cystitis (*See* CYSTITIS). Treatment may be by pessaries or oval tablets depending on the type of germ.

Vaginal infection can of course occur at any time of life and a variety of germs like monilia (thrush) and trichomonas (T.V.) as well as those of venereal disease may be the cause. Your family doctor can help with all of these infections although if you have risked venereal infection by casual sexual contact it is probably wise to go straight to a V.D. clinic. A discharge due to vaginitis can generally be distinguished from normal secretion by associated irritation or odour. A common cause of very offensive discharge is a retained tampon. Little girls are prone to vaginitis for, like their grannies, they too have low oestrogen levels. Persistent soreness and discharge in a child needs medical advice as apart from other considerations it may be due to the introduction of a "foreign body" such as a bead. Threadworms are another possible cause.

Varicocele. (*See* VARICOSE VEINS)

Name of a collection of dilated blood vessels in the scrotum – similar to varicose veins, and usually not serious. Sometimes a varicocele will cause aching and discomfort, when it can be removed by a small operation, or a suspensary bandage will sometimes meet the case. The condition may largely improve by the age of 30 when the bandage can be discarded.

A varicocele which may be associated with infertility can be treated by operation; it is safe and most men would prefer this to a bandage.

Varicose Veins.

Blood which circulates to the legs returns to the heart in thin-walled vessels. Some of these vessels, or veins, run just beneath the skin, and contain valves which prevent the blood from running down again into the leg. These surface veins connect with the deep veins in the leg by veins known as perforators.

In adults, the valves in the surface and perforating veins may become weakened, and the walls of the veins have to bear increased pressure. In consequence the veins become swollen and twisted, i.e. *varicose*. If the condition is left untreated the nourishment of the skin by fresh blood is interfered with, and an ulcer may occur (a *varicose ulcer*) which can be difficult to heal.

Some varicose veins can be treated by injection, which is simple. The swollen veins are emptied of blood by elevating the leg, and it is firmly bandaged afterwards and the patient is advised to walk at least three miles a day. This is to encourage blood flow in the more important *deep* veins which are in the muscles of the leg. The bandage can usually be discarded after about six weeks but it is good to continue the walking exercises and avoid standing for long periods. The small injection causes the vein to shrivel and disappear.

Some varicose veins can be controlled by supporting stockings or tights but these must be put on first thing in the morning before rising (i.e. before the surface veins become engorged by gravity). They must also extend well above the site of the highest varicose vein. It is no good wearing a knee length stocking when there are varicose veins in the thigh; this can make matters worse. An operation may be required to tie off or remove the vein. If a varicose ulcer has developed, it is essential that these veins should receive treatment – perhaps removal of associated veins; in addition the leg will need special dressings and compression bandaging while the ulcer heals. Your doctor can arrange for the community nurse to do this. The earlier treatment for varicose veins can be started the better. One aims to avoid complications and persistent leg pain. Varicose veins commonly occur during pregnancy and the best treatment is to wear supporting maternity tights and keep the feet up as much as possible. They usually recede quite a bit after the pregnancy is over.

Vasectomy. (*See* CONTRACEPTION)

Venereal Disease (*V.D.*) (*See* GONORRHOEA, SYPHILIS, *and* N.S.U.)

Verruca. (*See* WART)

Vertigo.
A sensation of movement of the surroundings; this can be rotational or horizontal and vertical. It is due to some temporary disturbance of the inner ear perhaps infection or upset in circulation. Tablets such as Stemetil or Serc are often helpful. A combination of tinnitus, vertigo and hearing loss is known as Menière's disease. Treatment is by the above tablets or occasionally by operation. (*See* GIDDINESS)

Virus.
Many germs which cause disease in man can be seen under a powerful light microscope. In one group the germs are so tiny they cannot be seen except under the modern electron microscope. These are known as viruses and unfortunately there is very little specific treatment for virus infections. Virus infections tend to be complicated by bacterial infections at a later stage so that antibiotics may help to treat and prevent complications.

Vitamin. (*See article on page* 9)

Vomiting. (Sickness)
Vomiting is brought about by contraction of the stomach muscles which empties the stomach of its contents. The

commonest cause is irritation by unsuitable or excessive food. Vomiting helps to protect the body from the unpleasant effects that might follow if the offending material were not eliminated. Examples are the eating of green apples by children, or excess alcohol by adults. Germs and food poison result in vomiting, and sometimes it is associated with disease of the stomach or intestines, for example GASTRIC or DUODENAL ULCER. Vomiting is controlled by a part of the brain, and if this becomes irritated sickness may occur without the stomach itself being irritated. This type is seen in MIGRAINE and in a variety of feverish illnesses. The vomiting in TRAVEL SICKNESS is also due to reflex irritation of the "vomiting centre". Vomiting also can be due to psychological reasons.

In the treatment of vomiting remember children tend to vomit more readily than adults and often get rid of phlegm in this way. If there is an obvious cause (e.g. too rich food and drink) the sickness will pass and need not alarm. Vomiting which occurs for no apparent reason or persists or is accompanied by pain should receive medical advice. "Coffee ground" appearance of the vomited material may indicate blood requiring urgent medical attention. (*See* HAEMATEMESIS)

W

Wart. *(Verruca)*

Small, hard outgrowths from the skin. They usually occur on hands, and feet, are mildly contagious, and may spread on the same person, or to another. Caused by a virus, warts sometimes disappear after months or years but because of the danger of spreading are best treated. Compound W or Verrugon can be applied daily to "burn" away the warts. The compounds must not contact normal skin which they will burn. Warts on the sole of the foot become compressed and painful and are usually known by their "correct" name of verrucae. Similar compounds will eventually cure but can be time consuming. People with verrucae are excluded from public swimming pools and should not take part in communal barefoot activities. Chiropodists will treat verrucae and most Local Authorities run Verruca Clinics for treatment. Stubborn verrucae can be frozen with carbon dioxide "snow" in hospital out-patients clinics (a doctor's letter is necessary).

Wax.

Soft wax is normally produced in the canal which leads to the ear drum. Some people produce more than others and if wax accumulates it becomes dry and hard and may reduce hearing or irritate. It can be removed by a doctor or nurse by syringing with warm water: it helps if the patient uses some softening drops such as Cerumol or Waxsol for a few days before the syringing. It is folly to try to remove the wax by syringing or poking things into the ear yourself, since the delicate ear drum may be damaged.

Wen. (*See* CYST)

White Leg.

Popular name for a condition which sometimes occurs in women after confinement. Fortunately it is rare due to the practice of encouraging women to get up and about as soon as reasonably possible after the birth. It is due to a blood clot in the circulation of the leg (*See* THROMBOSIS), and the limb becomes white, swollen and often painful. The condition needs urgent medical attention as the blood clot may dislodge from the leg and come to rest in the lung (*See* EMBOLISM). Special drugs can be given to diminish clotting and may be continued for six to twelve weeks. Blood tests at weekly intervals are needed to monitor the degree of "blood thinning".

Whitlow.

Infection in the fold of tissue on either side of the fingernail – it can spread below the nail. Bathing in hot salt water may bring the infection to a head and allow pus to escape. If infection persists and spreads below the nail antibiotics and perhaps drainage of pus may be necessary. (*See* FINGER, SEPTIC.)

Whooping Cough.

A specific infectious illness, usually in children, caused by a bacillus. The disease often occurs in epidemics and may be grave in babies. A second attack is unusual, but older children or adults, who have escaped infection, sometimes catch the disease. The germs are spread through the air, and the incubation period (*See* QUARANTINE; is usually about a fortnight. Early symptoms resemble those of a "cold", but continue longer with an increasing cough. The characteristic "whoops" do not usually develop for about two to three weeks. There is severe coughing which the child is unable to control; the face may become blue, and finally the breath is drawn in with a "whoop". These attacks occur a variable number of times a day, depending on the severity of infection, and are often troublesome at night. They are frequently followed by vomiting. This acute stage lasts from one to three weeks and although antibiotics such as erythromycin are usually prescribed it is not certain how far these are effective in shortening the illness.

Due to scares about damage being caused by whooping cough vaccine there have been large numbers of unvaccinated children at risk for the first time in twenty-five years in the U.K. The result has been a great increase in the illness. Young doctors have been seeing cases for the first time and it is too early as yet to be sure of the results of antibiotics in treating this unpleasant condition. Intensive care in hospital may be necessary in treating the very young who may develop complications such as pneumonia.

Advice should be sought at the first signs of spasmodic cough in a child in case it may be whooping cough. The child is rested during the feverish stage of the illness but may be allowed up when he is feeling better and more lively. If a child wants to be up and about he is usually well enough to do so. He should not return to school or playgroup until at least three weeks after the cough has stopped – assuming he feels well and energetic. He should have a final check from the doctor to make sure that the chest is clear before returning to school and at least a week of convalescence including outdoor walks to make sure that cold air does not provoke more coughing spasms. A minor degree of cough may persist for weeks but provided the child is otherwise well and lively it can be ignored.

Immunization is offered free to babies, in the form of "Triple" vaccine (it also contains protection against diphtheria and tetanus) at three, five and eleven months. Whooping cough is serious and can permanently damage the lungs and brain in severe cases. There has recently been anxiety about occasional harmful effects of the vaccine in causing brain damage. Epidemics of whooping cough cause much more damage then the vaccine but if you are worried about triple vaccine discuss this with your doctor. An alternative vaccine containing only the diphtheria and tetanus components can be given instead.

Womb. (*See* BIRTH *and* CERVIX)

Worms.

Various worms can inhabit the body. Their eggs are usually eaten accidentally with food and hatch in the digestive tract where they live on their host's food. Small worm infestation seldom causes serious symptoms; but *tapeworms* can take a considerable proportion of the nourishment and may disturb general health, and cause such side effects as anaemia or loss of weight. One of the common worms in this country is the *thread worm,* which usually affects children. It appears in the stools from time to time, where it resembles short pieces of white thread. If suspicious watch for it. It may cause itching, particularly at night, since the worms come out onto the buttocks to lay their eggs. This irritation may be a cause of bed-wetting and in girls scratching can lead to secondary infection and vaginal discharge.

Threadworms can be cured easily by appropriate medicines, such as Antepar and Vanquin, but reinfection must be guarded against. If itchy, children will tend to scratch their buttocks at night so thumb suckers and nail biters are particularly at risk from reinfection. Nails should be cut short and scrupulous hygiene observed. Everyone should have their own face cloths and towel which should be boiled after use. If one member of a family has threadworms treat the whole family. Other types of worm may infest man, but they are not common in the U.K. Any persistent itching round the buttocks or the appearance of worms in the stools should be reported to your doctor.

X

X-Rays.

Invisible to the eye, they resemble light rays in many ways but have greater penetration. Just as light will pass through glass X-rays pass through the tissues of the body. In common with light rays, X-rays can change a photographic plate which property makes them useful in medicine. By shining X-rays through a part of the body we can photograph the shadows they cast, and X-ray photographs reveal a number of internal disorders such as bone fractures which cannot otherwise be seen. The internal structure of the stomach and intestines can be studied by giving the patient an opaque substance such as barium sulphate to swallow (it can also be given as an enema into the lower bowels). The barium fills all the cavities and crevices of the intestines showing up ulcers or tumours. Another substance is given when the gall bladder is to be studied. A radio-opaque dye can be injected into the blood and photographed as it is filtered through the kidneys. This outlines the kidneys and bladder, demonstrates damage, stones or tumours and to some extent indicates the efficiency of the organ in filtering. Apart from the discovery of disease, or diagnosis, X-rays are useful in treating a number of conditions. In large doses the rays damage, and may kill cells, and this may be very useful in some cancers or in certain blood diseases.

PUBLISHER'S NOTE

In the case of many diseases and conditions, there exist organizations or societies devoted to research or to helping sufferers. Your Family Doctor should be able to put you in touch with these.

The rate of scientific progress in the medical field is very fast, and this book is constantly revised and improved in order to keep it up to date with the latest findings. The Publishers would be pleased to hear from any reader who would like to comment on any of the contents of the book.

INDEX